"With this remarkable work of scholarship, Van Haute and Westerink continue their pathbreaking project of making visible a largely unfamiliar Freud. Their meticulous readings demonstrate not only the historical and conceptual significance of the first edition of *Three Essays*, but also its astonishing relevance for contemporary debates about sex and gender."

—**Tim Dean**, *James M. Benson Professor in English, University of Illinois, Urbana-Champaign, USA*

"Philippe Van Haute and Herman Westerink reveal the multi-layered character of this text. Revealing a non-oedipal theory of sexuality in the 1905 edition and highlighting a theory of sexual pleasure and its potential for a radical critique of heteronormativity, they also remind us that it is us – our reading habits – that turn Freud into a monolithic thinker he has never been."

—**Daniela Finzi**, *Scientific Director of the Freud Museum Vienna*

"Van Haute and Westerink present their own systematic reading of Freud's text through the vicissitudes of its rewriting in no less than four successive re-editions from 1905–1924. What is at stake is the radicality of Freud's 1905 thesis of the polymorphous perverse nature of an infantile sexuality."

—**John Fletcher**, *Professor Emeritus, University of Warwick, Senior Research Associate, Psychoanalysis Unit, University College London*

"Intensifying rather than trying to iron out Freud's contradictions, Van Haute and Westerink allow the critical potential of the *Three Essays* to come to the fore, with the excavation of those (non-oedipal, pleasure-based and auto-erotic) elements that work in opposition to the heteronormative, functional conceptions of sexuality that still circulate today."

—**Stella Sandford**, *Professor of Modern European Philosophy, Kingston University, London*

READING FREUD'S THREE ESSAYS ON THE THEORY OF SEXUALITY

Sigmund Freud's 1905 *Three Essays on the Theory of Sexuality* is a founding text of psychoanalysis and yet it remains to a large extent an "unknown" text. In this book Freud's 1905 theory of sexuality is reconstructed in its historical context, its systematic outline, and its actual relevance.

This reconstruction reveals a non-oedipal theory of sexuality defined in terms of autoerotic, non-objectal, physical-pleasurable activities originating from the "drive" and excitability of erogenous zones. This book, consequently, not only calls for a reconsideration of the development of Freudian thinking and of the status of the Oedipus complex in psychoanalysis but also has a strong potential for supporting contemporary non-heteronormative theories of sexuality. It is as such that the 1905 edition of *Three Essays* becomes a highly relevant document in contemporary philosophical discussions of sexuality.

This book also explores the inconsistencies and problems in the original theory of sexuality, notably the unresolved question of the transition from autoerotic infantile sexuality to objectal adult sexuality, as well as the theoretical and methodological shifts present in later editions of *Three Essays*. It will be of great interest to psychoanalysts and those with an academic interest in the history of psychoanalysis and sexuality.

Philippe Van Haute is Professor for Philosophical Anthropology at Radboud University Nijmegen, the Netherlands, and Extraordinary Professor of Philosophy at the University of Pretoria, South Africa. He has published extensively on the relation between psychoanalysis and philosophy.

Herman Westerink is Associate Professor for Philosophy of Religion and Intercultural Philosophy at Radboud University Nijmegen, the Netherlands, and Extraordinary Professor at the KU Leuven, Belgium. He has published many books and articles on Freudian psychoanalysis, sexuality and religion.

The History of Psychoanalysis Series

Series Editors

Professor Brett Kahr and Professor Peter L. Rudnytsky

This series seeks to present outstanding new books that illuminate any aspect of the history of psychoanalysis from its earliest days to the present, and to reintroduce classic texts to contemporary readers.

Other titles in the series:

Corresponding Lives
Mabel Dodge Luhan, A. A. Brill, and the Psychoanalytic Adventure in America
Patricia R. Everett

A Forgotten Freudian
The Passion of Karl Stern
Daniel Burston

The Skin-Ego
A New Translation by Naomi Segal
Didier Anzieu

Karl Abraham
Life and Work, a Biography
Anna Bentinck van Schoonheten

The Freudian Orient
Early Psychoanalysis, Anti-Semitic Challenge, and the Vicissitudes of Orientalist Discourse
Frank F. Scherer

For further information about this series please visit www.routledge.com/The-History-of-Psychoanalysis-Series/book-series/KARNHIPSY

READING FREUD'S THREE ESSAYS ON THE THEORY OF SEXUALITY

From Pleasure to the Object

Philippe Van Haute and Herman Westerink

Routledge
Taylor & Francis Group
LONDON AND NEW YORK

First published 2021
by Routledge
2 Park Square, Milton Park, Abingdon, Oxon OX14 4RN

and by Routledge
52 Vanderbilt Avenue, New York, NY 10017

Routledge is an imprint of the Taylor & Francis Group, an informa business

British Library Cataloguing-in-Publication Data
A catalogue record for this book is available from the British Library

Library of Congress Cataloging-in-Publication Data
A catalog record for this book has been requested

ISBN: 978-0-367-64530-4 (hbk)
ISBN: 978-0-367-36430-4 (pbk)
ISBN: 978-1-003-12498-6 (ebk)

Typeset in Bembo
by Apex CoVantage, LLC

CONTENTS

ACKNOWLEDGMENTS

This book results from a larger project on *Three Essays* that has already produced several major publications. Parts of the first chapter of this book have already been published – in shorter versions and altered compositions – in the form of commentaries to translations and new editions of the 1905 *Three Essays* (Freud 1905a, 2015, 2017) and articles (Haute & Westerink 2016a, 2016b). Also, we should mention here the publication of two volumes – a first in which various authors explore aspects of the first edition of *Three Essays* (Haute & Westerink 2017) and a second that investigates the Dora case study and its relevance for Freudian theory (Finzi & Westerink 2018).

We would like to thank the many colleagues with whom we were able to discuss our thoughts and ideas on Freud's theory of sexuality at various meetings, symposia, and conferences over the past few years. Their comments contributed highly to our project. We would especially like to thank Ulrike Kistner for her reading and excellent translation of the 1905 *Three Essays* and the many productive conversations we had on the text. It was a privilege to work so closely with her. Also, we are very grateful for the meetings of the Freud Research Group and the many discussions with its members, Irene Berkel, Fons van Coillie, Monique David-Ménard, Jens De Vlemick, Daniela Finzi, Gilles Ribault, Ednei Soares, Beatriz Santos, Céline Surprenant, and Patrick Vandermeersch, on Freudian theory. In addition, we would like to explicitly thank our colleagues at the Center for Contemporary European Philosophy for their willingness to think through the project with us. We would like to thank Bob Vallier for the excellent correction work, Brett Kahr and Peter L. Rudnytsky for giving us the opportunity and honor to publish our book in the History of Psychoanalysis Series, and the Routledge editors Russell George and Alec Selwyn for guiding us through the publication process.

SERIES EDITOR'S FOREWORD

On December 12, 1904, Dr. Sigmund Freud, then forty-eight-and-a-half years of age, delivered a talk, "Über Psychotherapie" ("On Psychotherapy"), to colleagues in the Wiener Medizinisches Doktorenkollegium (Viennese Medical Doctor's College). As Freud would soon turn forty-nine years of age on May 6, 1905, he no doubt found himself much preoccupied with his own impending half-century.

In his presentation, Freud (1905f: 213) expressed concern that as patients approach or reach the age of fifty years, they begin to lose their mental "Plastizität" ("plasticity") and become, alas, less educable and, therefore, less suitable for psychoanalytical treatment. Needless to say, modern-day psychotherapists and psychoanalysts would question Freud's characterization of the older members of the population; and in more recent years, colleagues have undertaken excellent work on the treatment of the elderly through traditional psychoanalytical means (e.g., King 1980; Coltart 1991; Aldrich 1994; Junkers 2006; Amos & Balfour 2007; Davenhill 2007). One cannot help but wonder whether Freud made his observation about the dangers of aging, at least in part, because of his own encroaching birthday, just over a year away.

Thus, with his fiftieth anniversary in the offing, Freud no doubt worked extremely diligently to produce as many substantial contributions as possible throughout the year 1905, prior to his major birthday on May 6, 1906.

Throughout 1905, Freud (1905a) worked like a Trojan to complete several major monographs: first, a substantial text entitled *Der Witz und seine Beziehung zum Unbewussten* (*Jokes and Their Relation to the Unconscious*), which, we suspect, appeared in print in the spring of that year, as Freud dated his own personal copy – currently preserved in the safe of the Freud Museum London – May 22, 1905. Some months later, during the autumn, he published a seminal case history in two parts about an hysterical patient known as Dora in a medical periodical, the

Monatsschrift für Psychiatrie und Neurologie (*Monthly for Psychiatry and Neurology*) (Freud 1905d, 1905e).

But, perhaps most profoundly of all, Freud (1905b) produced yet another book; namely, the *Drei Abhandlungen zur Sexualtheorie* (*Three Essays on the Theory of Sexuality*), which would become one of the most important tomes in the entire history of international psychology. Though only eighty-three pages in length, this short text broke considerable new ground and provided the foundation for an entirely fresh, bold, and daring theory of human sexuality.

Although it would be unfair to describe Freud as the inventor of modern sexuality per se, he certainly created a new form of discourse in which erotic phantasy and behavior could be conceptualized more frankly and profoundly. From a sexological perspective, Freud followed in the footsteps of such authors as Professor Richard von Krafft-Ebing (1886), one of the most celebrated of German-speaking psychiatrists, best known for his remarkable work, *Psychopathia Sexualis: Eine klinisch-forensische Studie* (*Sexual Psychopathy: A Clinical-Forensic Study*), first published in 1886. Whereas von Krafft-Ebing's book reads like a chronicle of disgust, Freud's monograph strikes us as a much more libertarian, progressive, and honest work, explaining that non-procreative sexuality cannot be dismissed as merely the horrifying indulgences of the pathological and the perverse, but, rather, that every human being enjoys a complex sexual life, underpinned by infantile wishes and anxieties.

During the latter part of the nineteenth century, Richard von Krafft-Ebing's book attracted considerable attention and became, for many years, the gold standard work of reference about sexual crimes and oddities. Freud had reason to loathe von Krafft-Ebing and may have also harbored a wish to outdo him as Austria's leading sexologist, not least because the older physician had once shamed Freud publicly back in 1896, dismissing his contributions as little more than a "wissenschaftliches Märchen," or "scientific fairy tale" (Freud 1896a: 193). Consequently, although Freud would cite von Krafft-Ebing in his own book on sexuality published in 1905, he made only a few brief and not particularly significant references to the work of his senior colleague.

Sigmund Freud's classic study of sexuality has become a staple among psychoanalysts and psychotherapists worldwide, and it remains, to this day, a source of huge insight and inspiration that helps us to understand the nature of the erotic mind. I certainly could not have undertaken my own research on the sexual fantasies of British and American adults – more than 25,000 individuals in total – focusing on the traumatic childhood origins of sexual states of mind (Kahr 2007, 2008), without having spent years absorbing the insights first identified by Freud only months before his own fiftieth birthday.

But those of us who read the works of Sigmund Freud nowadays find ourselves confronted with a potentially serious problem. Mercifully, in spite of the tragic fact that the Nazis burned many of Freud's books in 1933, we still have innumerable editions of his many writings, not only in German and English but also in many other languages. Indeed, we have no shortage of Freud texts to which we may turn.

English-speaking readers who do not or cannot tackle Freud in German will, in all likelihood, have embraced the father of psychoanalysis through the wonderfully clear and accurate translations carefully supervised by James Strachey. However, in spite of the brilliance and authenticity of Strachey's fluid and readable rendering of the *Drei Abhandlungen zur Sexualtheorie* as the *Three Essays on the Theory of Sexuality* (Freud 1905c), many students and practitioners alike may not fully realize that Strachey's edition of Freud's work consists not only of an incorporation of the original 1905 version of the book but also of an amalgamation of the many additional passages and notes contained in the second edition of 1910, the third edition of 1915, the fourth edition of 1920, the fifth edition of 1922, the revised fifth edition of 1924, and the sixth edition of 1925. Although Strachey – a formidable translator – crisply delineated each addendum with appropriate scholarly notations, contemporary Freud enthusiasts will not readily be able to differentiate the original text of 1905 from the expanded version of 1925 with much ease. And while most Freudian students could not care less whether they immerse themselves in a first edition or a sixth edition, those of us who *do* wish to understand the development of Freud's theories over time and *do* yearn to study his contribution in a more serious and systematic way may find ourselves vexed or confused.

Thankfully, Professors Philippe Van Haute and Herman Westerink, two extremely meticulous researchers from Nijmegen in the Netherlands, have studied each edition of Freud's sexual masterpiece with microscopic skill and have provided a compelling and convincing narrative, explaining why one might benefit from reading the very first edition in its unedited form, underscoring how a careful investigation of Freud's tract, in its original incarnation, will shed tremendous light on the truly radical, revolutionary nature of his contributions, emphasizing the ways in which Freud embraced sexuality in a non-pathologizing and non-moralistic manner.

I shall not reveal the specificities of the remarkable detective work that has emerged from the extensive historical investigations of Professors Van Haute and Westerink, but I shall underscore that, as a result of reading this book, one will walk away far more knowledgeable about the precise nature of Freud's paradigm-shifting contributions to the theory of sexuality as well as the complex and intricate journey of theory construction that unfolds across the many revisions of this seminal text. I certainly have learned a great deal, and I thank the authors warmly for having written such an engaging book and for having reminded us that the "tidy" version of an updated Freud may not always be the most accurate or, indeed, the most original.

Professor Brett Kahr,
Series Co-Editor,
History of Psychoanalysis Series

References

Aldrich, C.K. (1994). Senior Patients, Senior Psychiatrists, and Senior Politicians, in George H. Pollock (Ed.), *How Psychiatrists Look at Aging,* Vol. 2, Madison, CT: International Universities Press, 79–90.

Amos, A. & Balfour, A. (2007). Couples Psychotherapy: Separateness or Separation? An Account of Work with a Couple Entering Later Life, in R. Davenhill (Ed.), *Looking into Later Life: A Psychoanalytic Approach to Depression and Dementia in Old Age*, London: Karnac Books, 75–89.

Coltart, Nina E.C. (1991). The Analysis of an Elderly Patient, in *International Journal of Psycho-Analysis* 72, 209–219.

Davenhill, R. (2007). Individual Psychotherapy, in Rachel Davenhill (Ed.), *Looking into Later Life: A Psychoanalytic Approach to Depression and Dementia in Old Age*, London: Karnac Books, 62–74.

Freud, S. (1896). Letter to Wilhelm Fliess. 26th April, in J.M. Masson & M. Schröter (Eds.), *Briefe an Wilhelm Fliess 1887–1904: Ungekürzte Ausgabe,* Frankfurt am Main: Fischer Verlag, 193–194.

Freud, S. (1905a). *Der Witz und seine Beziehung zum Unbewussten,* Vienna: Franz Deuticke.

Freud, S. (1905b). *Drei Abhandlungen zur Sexualtheorie,* Vienna: Franz Deuticke.

Freud, S. (1905c). *Three Essays on the Theory of Sexuality,* J. Strachey (Transl.), in J. Strachey, A. Freud, A. Strachey & A. Tyson (Eds. and Transls.), *The Standard Edition of the Complete Psychological Works of Sigmund Freud, Volume 7. (1901–1905). A Case of Hysteria. Three Essays on Sexuality and Other Works,* London: Hogarth Press and the Institute of Psycho-Analysis, 130–243.

Freud, S. (1905d). Bruchstück einer Hysterie-Analyse. [Part I], in *Monatsschrift für Psychiatrie und Neurologie* 18, 285–309.

Freud, S. (1905e). Bruchstück einer Hysterie-Analyse. [Part II], in *Monatsschrift für Psychiatrie und Neurologie* 18, 408–467.

Freud, S. (1905f). Über Psychotherapie, in S. Freud (Ed.) (1906), *Sammlung kleiner Schriften zur Neurosenlehre aus den Jahren 1893–1906,* Vienna: Franz Deuticke, 205–217.

Junkers, G. (2006). Editor's Preface, in G. Junkers (Ed.), *Is it Too Late? Key Papers on Psychoanalysis and Ageing. Papers in* International Journal of Psychoanalysis *Key Papers Series,* London: Karnac Books, xi–xxii.

Kahr, B. (2007). *Sex and the Psyche,* London: Allen Lane/Penguin Books, Penguin Group.

Kahr, B. (2008). *Who's Been Sleeping in Your Head? The Secret World of Sexual Fantasies,* New York: Basic Books/Perseus Books Group.

King, P. (1980). The Life Cycle as Indicated by the Nature of the Transference in the Psychoanalysis of the Middle-Aged and Elderly, in *International Journal of Psycho-Analysis* 61, 153–160.

Krafft-Ebing, R. von (1886). *Psychopathia Sexualis: Eine klinisch-forensische Studie,* Stuttgart: Verlag von Ferdinand Enke.

INTRODUCTION

Three Essays on the Theory of Sexuality is one of Sigmund Freud's most important, original, and well-known writings. First published in 1905, it soon attracted attention and eventually became a landmark text in the history of Freudian psychoanalysis and beyond. It was a relatively short text compared to the various contemporary studies on sexuality published by scholars in neurology, sexology, and psychiatry, as it comprised no more than eighty-three pages. The reference to "1905" and "contemporary" indicates the context of *Three Essays.* The text is intrinsically bound to other publications in the same period, such as "Fragment of an Analysis of a Case of Hysteria" (the Dora case) and *Jokes and Their Relation to the Unconscious,* and to the culmination – and revision – of theoretical thoughts on and clinical insights into the role played by sexuality in the etiology of the psychoneuroses, notably hysteria. One might expect that any systematic reading of the text would start from this fact. And yet literature on the theoretical developments in Freudian psychoanalysis in general and his theory on sexuality in particular show that this is seldom the case. The difficulty here lies in the fact that Freud reissued *Three Essays* four times over a period of two decades (1910, 1915, 1920, 1924), each time deleting some – very crucial – sentences and concepts and adding long sections, paragraphs, and footnotes in which he presented in detail the theoretical "progress" that had been accomplished since the previous edition. One finds that Freud inserted large paragraphs on the drive and libido theory, the child's sexual researches, the phases of development of the sexual organization, narcissism, the diphasic object choice, the influence of phylogenetic material, and – in a few scattered footnotes – the Oedipus complex. The result of this was that the final version of 1924 was almost forty pages longer than the original edition, and it was this 1924 text that became the "officially approved" one; that is, the version taken up in the well-known collections of his writings (*Gesammelte Werke* and *Standard Edition*) as the publication coded "1905." This 1905 text, however, is in a sense a missing object to which every Freud scholar refers often without recognizing its "absence" from the standard collections of writings. This absence is not merely metaphorical – it is a fact. Until a few years ago (Freud 2015), the German 1905 edition was hardly accessible because very few original copies remained and only one almost unnoticed reprint was available (Freud 2005). The first English translation of the first edition has only very recently – in 2016 – been published, thus making the 1905 edition available for the first time in its own composition and reasoning (Freud 1905a).[1]

The absence of the 1905 edition of *Three Essays* has huge implications on various levels. These implications first of all concern any systematic reading of and reflection on the text itself. One might be tempted to take Freud's own statement in the preface to the 1910 edition as a guideline: "what was imperfect may be replaced by something better." From this perspective, the 1924 edition could be read as the "better" version in the sense that it articulates the "most complete" theory – and for this reason it would therefore also justifiably be the "officially approved" theory. By this reasoning, one likely assumes that the first version of the text is not complete when compared to every subsequent version – that is to say, either it has major deficiencies and leaves (too) many open questions unanswered and problems unsolved or it is in need of more profound theoretical substantiation and argumentation underpinning the first intuitions and explorations. The first version thus tends to become something like a draft, a first sketch of and outline for later versions. The various editions of the text would supposedly show continuity through the further clarification and systematization of ideas. The often not very hidden premise would then be this: *Three Essays* develops progressively into the "better" version, and this runs parallel to the steady advancements in psychoanalytic theory, methods, and practice.

This book presents a systematic reading of the first and various later editions of *Three Essays*.[2] This means making the "absent" theory of sexuality present again, not by considering the 1905 edition as a text that is less complete in comparison to the subsequent versions but by showing that the first and various later versions are different texts presenting different theories. The "absent" text is an "other" text – the 1905 theory of sexuality is fundamentally different from the later versions in which Freud indeed inserts new theoretical material and approaches that produce a different, redefined theory on sexuality. In other words, essential parts of the theory of infantile and adult sexuality as Freud presents these in inserted sections, paragraphs, and footnotes in the later editions of the text are virtually absent in the 1905 first version.

Our reading of the first and later editions of *Three Essays* also has implications for the view of the history of Freudian psychoanalysis. What does it mean to say that the later inserted material – for example, the sections on the drive and libido theory, the phases of development of the sexual organization, and the diphasic object choice or the few references to the Oedipus complex – is absent from the 1905 edition? Should we conclude from this that Freud felt uncertain in 1905 about the status of intuitions he had been developing since he had – allegedly – abandoned his seduction theory ten years before and had engaged himself in a productive self-analysis? If that were the case, the "absent" theoretical material might be considered already potentially or latently present like a hidden "truth" behind the text and between the lines – a truth that would also be the key to the interpretation of the text, i.e., to an oedipal reading of the text.

This book provides a historically and systematically contextualized reading of the first and later editions of *Three Essays* that explores the central concepts and compositions of ideas. Regarding the historical aspect, it is a fact that Freud's text connects to a body of literature in psychiatry, neurology, and sexology from the late nineteenth century. In this context, the 1905 edition of *Three Essays* marks an important shift. Until 1905, Freud had mainly expressed his ideas within the conceptual framework of neurology. In *Three Essays*, he adopts for the first time – and systematically – the conceptual framework of psychiatry and sexology. This includes, for example, a shift from a theory of affects toward a theory of the drives. Until 1905, Freud's conceptual framework, as he had developed it in his studies on hysteria, neurasthenia, and anxiety neurosis in the 1890s, mainly revolved around notions such as impulse (*Reiz*), endogenous excitation, affect, and psychic energy – concepts developed from his background in neurology. The concept of *Trieb* had not been part of that framework. It was in *Three Essays* that Freud first elaborated this concept in line with the contemporary psychiatric and sexological literature. Regarding the more systematic context, the 1905 *Three Essays* can be seen as Freud's last major text on hysteria, and for that reason it is closely related to the Dora case (also published in 1905) and to all previous writings on hysteria.

Notably, our reading of the first edition will reveal that many of the concepts and constructs generally considered fundamental to psychoanalytic theory had not yet been defined or even introduced at the time of its publication. With regard to this first edition, the central thesis in our book is that Freud develops a non-oedipal theory of infantile sexuality; that is, a theory that in principle cannot be articulated or translated in oedipal terms. In 1905, Freud had not yet articulated his theory of the Oedipus complex, nor had he focused his attention on the obsessional neurotic problematic of love, hate, ambivalence, identification, conscience, and guilt that would lead him to identify this complex. He had not yet formulated a theory of the drives, nor had he introduced his theory of narcissism, in which he would express his views on the association between the drive economy and object relations. Moreover, he had not committed himself to a developmental approach in thinking about the relation between early childhood, puberty, and adulthood. These and other later inserted elements contain new material that fundamentally disrupts the original ideas and perspectives on infantile sexuality as being composed of polymorphous perverse, autoerotic, and non-objectal pleasurable activities. Of course, the two decades between the first and last editions of *Three Essays* had seen fundamental changes in Freud's thinking. He was well aware of this fact: "[r]eaders of my *Three Essays on the Theory of Sexuality* will be aware that I have never undertaken any thorough remodelling of that work in its later editions, but *have retained the original arrangement* and have kept abreast of the advances made in our knowledge by means of interpolations and alterations in the text. In doing this, it may often have happened that *what was old and what was more recent did not admit of being merged into an entirely uncontradictory whole*" (Freud 1923a: 141, emphasis ours). Indeed, we will illustrate that the final "officially approved" edition of 1924 is in many respects contradictory and inconsistent; or, in other words, any of Freud's presumed attempts to solve problems, answer open questions, or resolve inconsistencies present in the 1905 edition resulted in creating new ones. And, as we will show, this was inevitable exactly because he maintained the original arrangement of the text; that is, three essays in which two distinct regimes of sexuality – the infantile and the adult – are presented.

In Chapters 2 and 3, in which the various later editions of *Three Essays* are explored, the central hypothesis is the following: whereas the 1905 theory of (infantile) sexuality presents a radical critique of the contemporary functional and heteronormative perspective on sexuality by highlighting the polymorphous perverse and autoerotic character of sexuality, the later editions reveal a progressive undermining of the radical character and critical potential of the first version. This critical potential, of course, first of all concerns his discussion with his contemporaries in the field of late nineteenth-century *scientia sexualis*, notably Freud's deconstruction of the sharp distinction between the normal and natural organization of sexuality in the service of preservation of the species on the one hand and the perversions as abnormal, pathological aberrations on the other. The fact that Freud in 1905 presents a non-oedipal theory of sexuality is of crucial importance for determining its further critical potential. If – as we will argue in this book – the steady oedipalization of Freudian theory, in combination with a turn to a developmental approach, can be seen as a "return" to the heteronormative views of his contemporaries, then the critical potential of the 1905 edition also concerns Freudian theory itself. One can read "with Freud against Freud" and consequently against the post-Freudian psychoanalysis that was preoccupied with object-relations, the Oedipus complex, and the conceptualization of "good enough" family structures. Our "return" to the first edition of *Three Essays* thus raises questions as to the nature and purpose of any "return to Freud." To which Freud does one return when one argues for such a return? And what are its implications?

In this light, there is another critical potential of the 1905 theory of sexuality. Freud's view of the polymorphous perverse pleasures and the need for variation that characterizes sexual activities does not merely contrast with the views held in late nineteenth-century *scientia sexualis*: the relationship is more complicated. As Foucault has argued, one cannot understand nineteenth-century *scientia sexualis* if one does not recognize its continuity with a Christian hostility toward a variety of pleasurable sexual activities (hence, the disavowal of "the use of pleasure") and the promotion of marriage in its normalizing function for the organization of sexuality – the heterosexual partner choice with the aim of the production and raising of children. In other words, *Three Essays* is also a key text in any history of sexuality, and Freud unintentionally refers to this long history when using the concept of libido in the opening sentences of the text (Freud 1905a: 1). More explicit ideas can be found in the following years, when Freud distinguishes cultural stages in the history of sexual morality, arguing that there is a development from relative sexual freedom toward intensified limitation and juridical regulation of sexuality in the service of reproduction (Freud 1908b: 189). This parallels another development Freud articulates in the 1910 edition of *Three Essays*: "the most striking distinction between the erotic life of antiquity and our own no doubt lies in the fact that the ancients laid stress upon the instinct [drive] itself, whereas we emphasize its object" (Freud 1905c: 149). Following Foucault's ideas on the history of sexuality, one could argue that the term *libido* plays a vital role in this history, shifting meaning from lusts and appetites that ought to be tempered to obtain an optimum of pleasure and satisfaction in the leading of a good life (in Epicurean and Stoic thought) toward the – Augustinian – notion of a dominant, sinful sexual desire lurking in the dark corners of the soul and perverting all human activities (Foucault 2018). The libido is here something hostile and evil that needs to be either eradicated or domesticated in marriage; that is, bound to an object, not to obtain pleasure but with the aim of procreation.

What Foucault seems to have overlooked in his evaluation of psychoanalysis and its place in the history of sexuality is exactly Freud's 1905 theory of sexuality; that is, a theory of pleasure derived from autoerotic bodily sensations and ticklings. As Freud realized in the 1910 footnote we just mentioned, his conceptualization of infantile sexuality as non-objectal, autoerotic pleasure could be associated with the earlier version's stress on the drive and its relative freedom. In other words, what we find here in the first place is a theory of sexual pleasure and excitation, not a theory of sexual desire for an object that promises to provide enjoyment and that is hence bound not to physiological facticity but to a regulatory cultural ideal of heterosexuality – not "sex-desire," but rather "bodies and pleasures" ought to be the rallying point of a critical inquiry into the history of sexuality as a history of the conditions of the emergence of forms of subordination (Foucault 1978: 157; see also Butler 1999). In his project regarding "a historical and critical study dealing with desire and the desiring subject" (Foucault 1985: 5), Foucault's interpretation of psychoanalytic thought largely depends on Lacan's "return to Freud." In this view, Freud presents a theory of desire and objects; that is to say, a theory that is always already to some extent oedipalized and hence contaminated with the aim of establishing a cultural structure (the nuclear family) as the normal organizational form of sexuality and of identifying a number of sexual tendencies as abnormal, "evil" aberrations (the perversions) (Westerink 2019; Martins 2019).

This reference to Foucault's project regarding a history of sexuality provides us with a clearer view of what is at stake in our reading of the first and later editions of *Three Essays*. How does Freud redefine sexuality; resituate the perversions; define the relation between pathology and normality; conceptualize the body, its drives, pleasures, and excitations; and view the relation between human constitution (nature) and culture? And what would be the relevance and actuality of the 1905 edition of *Three Essays* for contemporary thought on sexuality, pleasure, perversion, pathology, and normality? Clearly, Freud's 1905 theory of sexuality resonates with the writings of Foucault and others such as Gilles Deleuze and Judith Butler – and with queer theory in its potential for developing a psychoanalytic metapsychology that escapes the heteronormativity that has characterized post-Freudian psychoanalysis up to now and that instead takes its starting point in the excitable body.

But, moreover, does Freud present a full-fledged subversive theory of sexuality in *Three Essays*? We have already mentioned the inconsistencies and ambiguities, which will be more thoroughly discussed in this book, and we have also pointed at the "return" of the functional perspective in the third essay on puberty and adult sexuality. Freud struggled not only with the inner coherence of his depiction of infantile sexuality and the limitations of the model of hysteria but also with thinking through the transition from infantile to adult sexuality while remaining bound to a cultural morality in which several implications of his ideas were actually unthinkable. Our reading of the various editions shows how productive these problems and open ends in fact were and can be. Taking his starting point in the model of hysteria for the inquiries into the human sexual constitution, Freud soon felt obliged to fundamentally engage with metapsychological questions concerning the drives, the relation to objects and to reality, aggression, ego formation, etc. This soon led him beyond the model of hysteria and its limitations. The study of other psychopathologies that were supposed to shed light on existing problems in fact produced new questions that needed answering. In short, our reading of the various editions of *Three Essays*, in its significance for contemporary psychoanalysis and philosophical anthropology, can be interpreted to a certain extent as a reconstruction of developments within Freudian thought up to 1924. However, since we confine ourselves to a reading of the various editions of *Three Essays*, our analyses of evolutions in Freudian psychoanalysis will necessarily be limited to the themes and issues that pertain to the theory of sexuality as presented in *Three Essays*.

Notes

1 The oldest version of *Three Essays* available in English is the 1910 edition translated by Abraham Brill. This version, however, is hardly ever referenced in literature.

2 Hence, this research is in line with, for instance, the work of Lydia Marinelli and Andreas Mayer on the different editions of *Die Traumdeutung* (Marinelli & Mayer 2003) and Ulrike May's re-reading of the various versions of *Jenseits des Lustprinzips* (May-Tolzmann 2015b). In showing the multi-layered character of Freud's texts, these readings allow us to understand these texts as a field of mutually related questions and problems that remain relevant for us today, rather than as a set of definitive answers that belong to history.

1

HYSTERIA AND SEXUALITY

Introduction

In this chapter, we will contextualize and reconstruct the various aspects of Freud's 1905 theory of sexuality. Such contextualization, both historical and systematic, is necessary since *Three Essays* can only be properly understood when situated against the background of developments in contemporary neurology, sexology, and psychiatry and in relation to other texts and projects Freud was working on around 1905. This approach will make it possible to identify both the continuity and radicality of the 1905 *Three Essays* relative to an existing body of literature and thought. With regard to the reconstruction of the content of the text, we will show that in 1905, Freud clearly distinguished between two regimes of sexuality. On the one hand, we find infantile sexuality, which is described in terms of autoerotic, polymorphous perverse sexual activities without object or specific aim – activities that cannot be described in functional terms. On the other hand, Freud formulates his ideas on sexuality as it becomes organized in puberty. Here, the experience of pleasure is still an important element but now only within a structure in which "normal" sexuality is characterized by a heterosexual object choice with the final aim of reproduction. This distinction of regimes not only has important implications but also raises several questions and problems that force Freud to reconsider his original ideas in the later versions of the text.

Studies in sexuality

Our point of departure is linked to an issue introduced on the very first page of *Three Essays*: its place within the body of work on sexuality, perversion, and pathology established in late nineteenth-century psychiatry, neurology, and sexology. Does Freud continue the modes of reasoning and conceptual frameworks presented in the literature he refers to in the first endnote of the text – the major writings of Richard von Krafft-Ebing, Havelock Ellis, Albert Moll, Iwan Bloch, and others from the 1880s and 1890s and the contemporary literature published in the first years of the twentieth century; for example, in Magnus Hirschfeld's *Jahrbuch für sexuelle Zwischenstufen*? Or does he develop something radically new – so new that the relation to these predecessors must be described in terms of a radical break? It is part of Freud's rhetorical strategy in the first pages of *Three Essays* to distance himself from the established body of thought on sexuality. Eminent predecessors are reduced to a footnote in a text that presents itself as opposed to "popular opinion" and "poetic fable" (Freud 1905a: 1). According to Freud, psychiatrists, neurologists, and sexologists had generally approached sexuality from a Darwinian perspective, focusing on the genital drive (*Geschlechtstrieb*[1]) as the manifestation of the reproductive instinct in the service of the preservation of the species.[2] From this perspective, which underscored the functionality of the human drives, sexuality had its analogy in hunger as the expression of the need for ingestion in the service of self-preservation. Within this scheme, Freud identifies a number of mistaken views on sexuality; namely, that it is absent in childhood, gains momentum only in puberty after the sexual organs have come to full maturation, and aims at procreative sexual acts with heterosexual partners.

No doubt Freud is referring here to some key aspects of the contemporary scientific and societal consensus on the nature of sexuality. In the opening passages of *Psychopathia Sexualis* (1886), Krafft-Ebing had stated that sexuality ought to be defined in terms of its natural function in the service of reproduction. This reproduction should not be regarded as the result of individual sexual preferences, but as the necessary and normal expression of a strong natural instinct for the preservation of the mental and physical capacities of the individual (Krafft-Ebing 1886: 1).[3] Formulated in this way, the Darwinian principles of the preservation of the individual and the species were closely related: preservation of the species was in fact motivated by the instinct of self-preservation. Reproduction was the means by which the life of the individual could be preserved beyond its intrinsic spatial and temporal limitations, as the individual's traits and capacities were preserved in future generations.[4] Sexuality was thus defined in purely functional terms as a means toward an end. It was reproduction in the service of preservation that defined normal sexual acts and the normal choice of sexual partners. Only procreative sexual acts were considered normal. This functional understanding of sexuality was the underlying conception for Krafft-Ebing's views on pathology in general and sexual perversions in particular. It was likewise this functional understanding of sexuality that determined his identification of abnormal sexuality, or, in Krafft-Ebing's words, the "anomalies of the sexual function"; that is, sexual deviations from the norm of reproduction (Ibid.: 32).[5] He distinguished four categories of such functional anomalies. The first category was paradoxia. This was either the manifestation of the genital drive in early childhood, as evidenced in masturbation (often causing degenerative neuroses or psychoses), or the remanifestation of the genital drive in old age, most often in relation to senility. Krafft-Ebing defines this anomaly in terms of the sexual organs not yet or no longer properly functioning. The second category was sexual anesthesia, or absence of the genital drive, which mostly resulted from psychic degeneration or from cerebral or other anatomical defects. The third category was hyperesthesia, or abnormally increased genital drive, which was most often found in adults with a neuropathic constitution, as manifested in neurasthenia or hysteria, for example. The fourth functional anomaly was the one Krafft-Ebing was most interested in: paresthesia, or sexual perversion. He presents the following definition of perversion: "[w]ith opportunity for the natural satisfaction of the sexual instinct, every expression of it that does not correspond with the purpose of nature – i.e., propagation – must be regarded as perverse" (Ibid.: 52–53). Every non-procreative manifestation of the genital drive is a perversion. It is this criterion of the natural function of the genital drive that links the four main perversions to each other. After all, sadism, masochism, fetishism, and inversion (soon further differentiated into homosexuality and bisexuality) have nothing essential in common beyond their non-procreativity. They are different sexual activities and interests in which sexual pleasure and satisfaction are obtained while detached from the natural instinct of reproduction (Davidson 2001: 75–76).

We find a similar train of thought regarding the relation between sexuality and reproduction in the writings of the Berlin neurologist and sexologist Albert Moll. Like Krafft-Ebing's, his work was an important point of reference in *Three Essays* and was recognized in the 1905 edition for its contribution to the scientific study of contrary sexual feeling (inversion) and infantile sexuality. In his book on the sexual libido (1898), Moll paid a lot of attention to the relation between the genital drive and reproduction. Reflecting on the basic principles of Darwinism, he argued that the sole function of the genital drive of men and women was procreation. In nature, heterosexuality is therefore the normal inherited disposition in service of what Moll calls "the principle of teleology" – reproduction (Moll 1898: 241ff). The individual development and feeling of sexuality were merely the subjective side of the objective reproduction instinct. All individual physiological and psychological sexual processes could be explained by this instinct. According to Moll, the genital drive was composed of two complementary impulses. The "detumescence impulse" was a natural urge that produced the transformation of the genitals (with the aim of ejaculation during coitus), including the increase of feeling in the genitals (with the aim of sexual satisfaction). The "contrectation impulse" paralleled the first and consisted of an inclination to gently approach, touch, and kiss a person of the opposite sex.[6] It was theories such as Moll's, in which the combination of physiological developments and mental processes (desire, attachment) during and after puberty was in the service of reproduction, that Freud called "poetic fables."

By opposing the "popular opinion," Freud distanced himself from an authoritative medical opinion shared by the main contemporary experts in the field of the scientific study of sexuality (Westerink 2009: 58ff). Before we take a closer look at Freud's 1905 theory of sexuality, however, we should put his relation to his predecessors in perspective. There are, after all, very good reasons not to regard Freud's work as radically opposing a whole body of medical thought on sexuality.

It is most important to recognize that Krafft-Ebing, Moll, and others paved the way for Freud's *Three Essays*. In fact, these scholars had anticipated many of his ideas, including first of all the conceptualization of sexuality as a prevailing natural drive that is also the most powerful force in cultural development, notably in social bonding and family life, morality, religion, and art (Krafft-Ebing 1886: 1–17). This conceptualization implied that the medical study of sexuality could never be limited to pathological deviations originating from inherited and degenerative dispositions. Even though Krafft-Ebing was primarily interested in the etiology of the perversions, he realized that his study of pathological sexual deviations contributed to a much broader insight into the role of human sexual impulses in culture and throughout history. This idea was a precursor to Freud's insight that any theory of sexuality would have a general anthropological dimension, and that the sexual drive and its sublimation were culturally productive. It was his predecessors who had put sexuality on the map as a fundamental aspect of both human nature and cultural life.

This broader view of sexuality and culture, together with the conceptualization of sexuality in terms of a "natural drive," imbued the writings of Freud's predecessors with a powerful emancipatory potential. This was evidenced not only in the writings of Krafft-Ebing and Moll but also and especially in the *Jahrbuch für sexuelle Zwischenstufen*. Here we find a marked tendency toward a critique of the criminalization of so-called sexual perverts. After all, when sexual pathology could no longer be thought of as resulting from perverse sexual acts and, conversely, perverse sexual acts were understood as originating from a neuropathic disposition, homosexuals could no longer be regarded as morally responsible for their sexual inclinations. Instead of having juridical procedures invoked against them, they should receive therapeutic treatment. This is a typical train of thought in the literature on sexual perversions (for example, Fuchs 1902). And although Freud does not devote himself to juridical issues in *Three Essays*, his text on cultural sexual morality written a few years later closely connects with such ideas on abnormal dispositions and the way society should deal with the variety of sexual urges and aims (Freud 1908b).

The second area in which earlier scholars anticipated Freud's ideas concerns the identification of the four basic types of sexual deviations: sadism, masochism, fetishism, and inversion. Krafft-Ebing had in fact invented the categories of sadism and masochism and had introduced them as two of the four fundamental forms of deviation from normal sexuality; that is, as non-procreative sexual activities. It was also Krafft-Ebing and Moll who had pioneered the concepts of homosexuality and pedophilia in the 1890s. It is fair to say that their Darwinian, functional approach led to the identification of these sexual perversions as the non-functional counterparts to normal sexuality. In the first of the three essays, on sexual aberrations, Freud approvingly identifies these four fundamental forms as the main sexual perversions. Nevertheless, as we will see later, Freud will strongly oppose the functional approach of his predecessors, which leads him to a fundamentally new perspective on the relation between pathology and normality. This brings us to the third development that paved the way for Freud's *Three Essays*.

Krafft-Ebing, Moll, and others had implicitly undermined their own basic assumptions regarding the opposition between sexuality and the perversions. Although they would never abandon the strict distinction between the normal sexual instinct and its perverse pathological deviations, both Krafft-Ebing and Moll increasingly shifted their attention toward the gradual differences between normal and abnormal. In Krafft-Ebing's *Psychopathia Sexualis*, this shift can already be detected in his views on hyperesthesia and paresthesia. When describing sadism, for example, he argues that the close relation between pleasure and cruelty is not specific to sadism or masochism but should in fact be regarded as originating from general human physiological and psychological characteristics, such as the opposition between the active male and passive female roles in sexual relations. He also recognized a close relation between certain aggressive acts (such as biting) and the nature of sexual excitation. The conclusion Krafft-Ebing drew undermined his basic assumptions. He writes: "[s]adism is thus nothing else than an excessive and monstrous pathological intensification of phenomena – possible, too, in normal conditions in rudimental forms – which accompany the psychical sexual life, particularly in males" (Krafft-Ebing 1886: 56). This definition of sadism is typical of what gradually becomes the predominant view of sexual deviations. Clinical case material shows that it is virtually impossible to make sharp qualitative distinctions between the normal and the pathological. Perversions like sadism can be seen as exaggerations and intensifications of normal sexual impulses and acts. In this context, Krafft-Ebing's views on sexual inversion also changed, notably in his studies on homosexuality. Although Krafft-Ebing and others never abandoned the paradigm of heterosexuality as the normal functional form of sexuality, new insights into homosexuality blurred the sharp distinction between masculinity and femininity (Ibid.: 188). Krafft-Ebing had again shown the way, suggesting that both innate and later, acquired homosexuality originated from what he identified as constitutional hermaphroditism or bisexuality. In one of his last articles, published in 1901, he stated explicitly that one should think of homosexuality as originating from what was essentially the human being's earliest embryonic disposition, hermaphroditism or bisexuality (Krafft-Ebing 1901: 8).[7]

Defining homosexuality in terms of an intermediate stage – recall the title of the above-mentioned *Jahrbuch* – was the next logical step. In the opening article of the year book's first volume (1899), the German sexologist Magnus Hirschfeld argued that homosexuality was indeed to be considered an intermediate form of sexuality that could be explained in terms of the gradual quantitative differences between men and women. Sexual deviations should preferably be interpreted in terms of variations within the larger spectrum of sexual gradations and individual expressions (Hirschfeld 1899). In other words, the clinical evidence showed that sexuality could not simply be differentiated or categorized in terms of a functional, natural instinct or its degenerative deviations. There were other aspects to be considered, most importantly the nature of sexual relations and choice of objects as well as sexual excitation, pleasure, satisfaction, and the individual's sexual needs. The German dermatologist and sexologist Iwan Bloch concluded the following from the vast amount of material on perversions and perversities (the latter term was coined by Krafft-Ebing to indicate the immoral sexual acts of normal people) and the observation that abnormal sexual conduct was present in all civilizations: sexual aberrations are not based on a neuropathic disposition but should instead be seen as generally human traits resulting from increased and intensified impulses (Bloch 1902: 6–7; Davidson 2001: 80–82). It was Freud who recognized this conclusion's revolutionary potential. Most sexual aberrations cannot be isolated from normal sexual life, and if sexual aberrations cannot be explained in terms of a neuropathic (inherited, degenerative) disposition, they can only be defined relative to a general human sexual disposition, described by Bloch and others in terms of an increase in or intensification of certain sexual impulses. Following this train of thought, in which the difference between normal and abnormal sexuality is merely quantitative, these increased sexual impulses inform us about not only pathologies but also, and more importantly, human nature in general. It is in this direction that Freud will proceed.

The dismissal of the functional approach to sexuality

Three Essays was written within the context of these developments in the scientific (medical, psychiatric) study of sexuality. But Freud immediately makes clear that he radically rejects the premises and paradigms his predecessors never fundamentally questioned, despite the fact that their clinical material provided many opportunities for them to do so. Dismissing the functional approach to sexuality as "fable," Freud starts where his predecessors had left off: the multitude of variations in human sexual life. To get a grip on these variations, Freud's own starting point is the distinction between the sexual object ("the person from whom the attraction on the other sex emanates") and the sexual aim ("the action impelled by the drive") (Freud 1905a: 1). By taking this starting point, Freud turned the approach of his predecessors upside down. They took the natural genital drive as the norm against which to identify pathological objects and aims and categorize the deviations. Freud, by contrast, wanted to study the sexual drive (*Sexualtrieb*) from the perspective of the variety of sexual objects and aims. Since the human sexual drive is not naturally organized by an inherent norm or according to some innate functional principle, there is indeed nothing but a variety of sexual activities and orientations in which there is no purely normal or absolutely abnormal sexuality. To explore this, let us take a closer look at the first of the three essays.

After the introductory remarks, Freud continues his chapter on sexual aberrations with a discussion of the deviations in relation to the sexual object. He primarily concentrates on homosexuality (inversion). Krafft-Ebing and others had been primarily interested in the question of the etiology of innate and acquired homosexuality, but Freud is not particularly interested in solving this riddle. Rather, he argues that inversion cannot be strictly separated from other forms of sexuality because of its wide spectrum of variations. He then continues with a critique of the most common explanations – that is, innateness, degeneration, and anatomical bisexuality (hermaphroditism) – and critically comments on the distinction between innate and acquired homosexuality (Ibid.: 3–6). Instead of formulating alternative approaches and answers to the question of etiology, Freud focuses on the observation of homosexuality in and outside of the clinical setting. These observations are as follows. First, homosexuality can be found in many persons who barely deviate from the common sexual norm. Second, homosexuality does not disturb a person's achievements. On the contrary, homosexuals are often highly advanced intellectually and morally. Third, while homosexuality can be found in all civilizations, the moral evaluation of homosexuality in different cultural contexts varies. From this he basically concludes that homosexuality as such cannot be classified as abnormal. This means that the established views on the distinction between normal and abnormal sexuality need to be reconsidered. Homosexuality cannot be interpreted in terms of a neuropathic deviation but should instead be seen as a modality of sexuality.[8] Freud also points to the fact that homosexuality can be viewed as a sexual aberration only with regard to its object – that is, the person from whom attraction proceeds (and one is subsequently attracted to) – not with regard to the sexual aims.

The most important conclusion Freud draws from his observations of homosexuality opens up a whole new theoretical realm, requiring a reconsideration of the relation between the sexual drive and the sexual object – there is no inherent object of an alleged natural sexual drive. "The genital drive," he writes, "is probably independent of its object initially, and its origin is likely not owed to the object's attractions" (Ibid.: 11). The idea that the sexual drive is independent of an object – that it expresses itself in a non-intersubjective way and does not in any way depend on the presence of an object – has far-reaching consequences for the understanding of sexuality in general. The implication is that all human sexuality is originally strictly non-functional. All references to the reproduction instinct, self-preservation, and preservation of the species implied the notion of the inherent object of the natural reproduction instinct.[9] Throughout *Three Essays*, this non-functional understanding of infantile sexuality is captured in the fundamental distinction Freud makes between the sexual drive (*Sexualtrieb*) and the genital drive (*Geschlechtstrieb*), with the latter indicating adolescent and adult sexuality that can again be understood in functional terms, as it had been in the writings of his predecessors. (This explains why Freud, in the just quoted statement, can link the genital drive to "its object" and "the object's attractions" when arguing that the sexual drive is in fact independent of an object.)

Freud's new radical starting point for the theory of sexuality had explosive potential within the psychoanalytic movement. This would be revealed at a meeting of the Wednesday Night Psychoanalytic Society in 1911, when Sabina Spielrein again defined the sexual drive as the "reproduction drive," with an inherent object (partner of the opposite sex) and aim (coitus) that "must" be used appropriately. "What troubles me most," Freud remarked, "is that Miss Spielrein wants to subordinate the psychological material to biological criteria" (Spielrein 1912: 98ff; Nunberg & Federn 1962: 335). Freud recognized the return of the old psychiatric style of reasoning within his own psychoanalytic movement. Spielrein allied herself with the functional view of sexuality, and she was not the only one. Carl Gustav

Jung – who was well acquainted with the psychiatric literature and concepts – officially approved of this position a year later when, in his critique of Freud's views on infantile sexuality, he proposed to define sexuality as the instinct for the preservation of the species or, in slightly different words, to regard normal sexuality as the manifestation of an original reproduction instinct and consequently to evaluate perversions as deviations from the normal development of sexuality (Jung 1912a: 144–145, 1912b: 127–128, 148–154). This implicit return to the style of reasoning of Freud's predecessors had a huge impact on the psychoanalytic movement and on Freud's thought in particular. The 1915 edition of *Three Essays* – the edition in which he added long passages on the theory of the drives, the libido theory (narcissism and object love), and infantile sexuality (oedipal thematic, object choice, developmental approach) – can be read as part of Freud's response to Jung (Vandermeersch 1991). But these newly added passages were hardly a defense of the 1905 theory of sexuality. The new passages in fact show that Freud dramatically changes his conceptualization of sexuality and, beyond this, the whole character of psychoanalytic theory at the moment he starts to rethink the nature of the sexual drives in relation to objects.

Perversion, the need for variation, and reaction formations

Having discussed deviations in relation to the sexual object, Freud turns his attention to sexual aims. His thoughts on this issue parallel his reasoning on the sexual object. Whereas Krafft-Ebing et al. represented the popular view in which coitus was seen as the normal sexual aim and all other sexual activities were regarded as perversions, Freud immediately states that these so-called perverse activities can actually be recognized as present in all normal sexual activities. According to Freud, the observation of sexual activities and relationships shows that the sexual aim is hardly ever limited to the genitals but involves the whole body as a surface of excitation and pleasure. It is not without irony and a sense of provocation that he raises the question of whether kissing (which he defines as the contact between the mucous membranes of the lips that constitute the entrance to the digestive tract) should be classified as a perverse act even though it is generally regarded as an aspect of every normal sexual relationship and therefore held in great esteem in civilized societies (Freud 1905a: 13). After all, like oral-genital activities, anal-genital activities, fetishism, sadomasochism, voyeurism, and exhibitionism, kissing involves body parts that do not belong to the sexual apparatus *sensu strictu*. He adds that the various sexual activities express a certain general human "need for variation" – a remark deleted from the 1920 edition onward (Ibid.: 14). Such a need for variation collides with cultural conventions on normal and abnormal sexual activities.

These conventions manifest themselves as disgust for certain sexual activities. Freud seems to suggest here that disgust is an expression of cultural morality, but in fact he argues that this is not the case. Drawing upon his studies of hysteria, he writes that shame and disgust are to be regarded as reaction formations. These reaction formations are psychic counterforces that are spontaneously constructed to repress the unpleasure that somehow results from sexual excitation. The crucial point here is that shame and disgust are seen as the "organically conditioned" limitations of the sexual drive, limitations reached without the involvement of external objects, norms, and principles. In 1906, Freud writes that his views on "organic sexual repression" were a crucial aspect of his theory of sexuality, which held that the essence of sexuality could be described in terms of pure physiological processes (Freud 1906: 278). An element of these physiological processes is organic repression, or reaction formations. Shame and disgust are therefore not the earliest manifestations of internalized cultural morality. The relation between the two is actually the other way around: cultural morality can only follow and impress "somewhat more clearly and deeply" the psychic lines "previously drawn organically" (Freud 1905a: 39). The 1905 edition of *Three Essays* was not the first time Freud had articulated this idea. As early as January 1896 he had written to Wilhelm Fliess that shame and disgust could not be explained as expressions of an interiorized cultural morality because clinical experience had shown that disgust could be overcome when the libido was strong enough to pursue its aims despite cultural norms. He deduced from this that there must be an independent source for the release of unpleasure, a source that makes the experience of disgust possible and empowers morality (Freud 1985: 163). He had returned to this issue in November 1897, arguing that the search for the source of normal sexual repression had led him to conclude that "something organic played a part in repression" – an idea he had found in one of Moll's writings (Ibid.: 280).[10] Exploring this idea, Freud argued that infantile sexuality was not yet organized through genital primacy but involved all erogenous zones, and maybe even the entire body surface, as sources of pleasurable sensations. In due time (puberty), and for some as yet unknown reason, the non-genital erogenous zones no longer produce sexual excitation, but rather unpleasure manifesting itself in disgust and shame. Although Freud could not deliver the answers to all the open questions on infantile sexuality, unpleasure, and repression, it was clear that repression could be thought of without reference to external influences and, hence, without reference to interiorized cultural morality. Infantile experience of pleasure and the later repression of the memories of these pleasurable experiences should be understood in terms of organic (biological) processes and subsequent psychic formations. It is such formations that provide the basic patterns and outline for the later internalization of cultural morality. Conversely, cultural morality will always be structured according to the psychic patterns that result from organic processes. Cultural morality follows organic processes, not the other way around.

According to Freud, disgust determines the identification of a certain sexual aim as perverse (Freud 1905a: 15). From the perspective of organic processes, this claim can be read according to the argumentation we have just described: disgust is an organically conditioned limitation of the sexual impulse ("Eek, dirty!"). This disgust is the psychic dam later strengthened by a culture's moral views. From the perspective of cultural morality, the qualification "perverse" is only a matter of consensus – that is, a nominal issue – because there is no natural norm for distinguishing between normal and abnormal sexual aims ("That dirty [thing you are doing] is perverse!"). The perversions can therefore only be defined in relation to what adults generally consider normal. Freud writes that certain perverse acts (licking shit or sexually abusing dead bodies) are so detached from normal sexual behavior that one should categorize them as pathological in contrast to normality (Ibid.: 21–22). Such detachment from normality is in fact the main criterion for identifying certain acts as perverse. But, more importantly, he stresses that most perverse sexual activities are part of normal sexual behavior – remember what we said about kissing – or can be found in persons who lead a perfectly normal life in all other respects. In fact, clinical evidence shows that most perversions are a composition of "pathological" and "normal" sexual aims (Meyer 2016: 70–71).

The main conclusion from this discussion of the variety of sexual acts is that the sexual drive is most likely put together using various components (Freud 1905a: 21). If sexual activities are composites, perhaps the source from which they spring (the sexual drive) is also a composite. It is from this conclusion that Freud makes the step toward a theory of the perverse polymorphous nature of infantile sexuality, the partial drives, and the erogenous zones. The ultimate conclusion to be drawn from Freud's views on the perverse polymorphous nature of infantile sexuality is already foreshadowed in his elaborations on the sexual aim: strictly speaking, there are no perversions since what we used to call perversions are in fact merely sexual activities in continuity with (through exclusiveness and fixation) the sexual disposition original to all human beings. The adjective *polymorphous* underscores the idea that infantile sexuality is not structured by any innate principle or order.[11]

Before we proceed to comment on the rest of the first essay, let us add two short remarks on sadism and masochism. In his discussion of the sexual aim, Freud is clearly guided by Krafft-Ebing's categorization of the perversions, which were authoritative in the field (Ibid.: 19). In the context of *Three Essays*, however, these two perversions are problematic, as they introduce two aspects of psychic life – aggression and pain – that are difficult to relate to infantile sexuality (De Vleminck 2013, 2017). As regards pain (and the experience of pleasure in pain), Freud writes that we should understand pain as a reaction formation, analogous to shame and disgust. Nevertheless, it is difficult to see how pain could be a psychic counterforce, and indeed, Freud does not and cannot explain his statement.[12] Later in the text he will mention compassion as a reaction formation against the pleasure of causing an object pain (Freud 1905a: 52), but of course this second statement does not answer the question of how pain can be a counterforce. Aggression and cruelty are equally difficult to understand. As we will see later, Freud will define infantile sexuality as the experience of pleasure through erogenous zones (corporeal excitation), drawing upon, for example, Moll's contrectation impulse, the inclination to gently approach, touch, and kiss an object. From this perspective, it is difficult to imagine aggression and cruelty as being "sexual" (pleasurable) or as components of the sexual drive. In other words, there are the questions of (1) the origin of aggressive and cruel impulses and (2) the relation between aggression and sexuality. Freud will argue that aggression and cruelty originate from a source other than the erogenous zones. The alliance between aggression/cruelty and sexual life is established relatively late in childhood (Ibid.). But this observation does not answer the two central questions. Freud therefore concludes that the perversions of sadism and masochism remain unsolved mysteries, and that the study of obsessional neurosis is most likely the key to understanding the sadistic component of the libido.[13] This is one of the reasons why Freud will turn his attention from hysteria to obsessional neurosis in the years after the first edition of *Three Essays*. In 1905, however, Freud's theory of sexuality is mainly formulated from the perspective of hysteria (or, more precisely, conversion hysteria). This brings us to Freud's discussion of the sexual drive in the psychoneuroses.

Hysteria as a model for understanding sexuality

Freud subsequently turns his attention to the psychoneuroses in general and hysteria in particular. He explains that hysteria provides the main model for the further conceptualization of sexuality (Ibid.: 24). We wish to highlight two important developments that led Freud to take hysteria as the model for the study of human sexuality. From the *Studies in Hysteria* in 1895 to the Dora case in 1905, Freud's clinical work had been mainly concerned with hysteria. Although his views on it had changed over the years, he had always remained true to an observation Jean-Martin Charcot had already communicated to him in the early 1880s: hysteria always involves the problematic of sexuality.[14] In his psychoanalytic practice, Freud had discovered that the origin of hysteria could be found in early childhood sexual experiences that had later been repressed from consciousness. The first major theory on the etiology of hysteria – the seduction theory (discussed further later) – was formulated in line with the general approach (the "popular opinion") that regarded neuroses as a deviation from "normality" because they originated from an "abnormal" (traumatic) moment in early childhood. When Freud started to question the exclusive etiological role of these accidental influences, he fell back on the most common interpretative scheme; namely, the influence of constitutional and hereditary factors. Nevertheless, there is a major difference between Freud and his predecessors, which can be seen in his 1906 claim that "in my theory the 'sexual constitution' took the place of a 'general neuropathic disposition'" (Freud 1906: 275–276). And in *Three Essays* he writes:

> [t]he conclusion now presents itself to us that there is indeed something innate lying at the basis of the perversions, but that it is *something innate in all human beings*, though as a disposition it may vary in its intensity and may lie dormant, waiting to be brought to the fore by life experiences.
>
> *(Freud 1905a: 32)*

In others words, Freud wants to explain hysteria or perversion as resulting not from an abnormal neuropathic disposition but from a general human sexual disposition,[15] and by taking this position he clearly distanced himself from the contemporary views on hysteria and the perversions.[16] The key questions in the study of hysteria were thus no longer "What is the specific accidental moment in the etiology of hysteria?" or "What is the neuropathic constitution from which we can explain hysteria?" but instead "How does hysteria originate from the general human sexual disposition?" and "What is sexuality?"

Freud's views on organic repression had played a key role in this change of perspective: (infantile) sexuality and repression could be explained in terms of general human physiological processes. The study of hysteria was apparently impossible without reference to a general human sexual constitution. Conversely, it could no longer be argued that the analysis of the psychopathologies should be limited to the field of pathology alone.[17] A redefinition of the relation between pathology and normality was required, and Freud provided one, arguing that pathologies can be seen as exaggerations and intensifications of normal sexual impulses and acts, keeping with a line of thought we have already identified in the clinical studies of Krafft-Ebing and others. In hysteria, we find constitutionally higher than average sexual energy, and we subsequently find repression of sexual impulses in excess of the normal measure (Ibid.: 25). Hysteria magnifies the general human physiological processes of sexuality, its repression, and the symptom formations that result from the unresolved conflict between the sexual impulses and repression.

Freud now takes a further important step: human life can best be studied from the perspective of a certain group of pathologies (namely, the psychoneuroses) because these pathologies display exaggerations of normal physiological and psychic processes and mechanisms and are not as estranged from normality as some other pathologies. If we are all to a certain extent hysterical, then hysteria can inform us about who we are. The study of pathology becomes what we – following Jacques Schotte (1990) – call the patho-analysis of human existence. Human nature as such can best and probably only be studied from the perspective of the psychopathological variations. In the 1905 *Three Essays*, hysteria is the variation that becomes the model for understanding all human sexuality and, beyond that, human nature (Haute 2005, 2013).

In principle, this perspective on pathological variations allows Freud to break away from the categorical approach that characterizes traditional and mainstream psychiatry. In the categorical approach, which interprets psychiatric taxa much as Carl Linnaeus orders plants in his *Species Plantarum*, one either belongs to a certain category or not, and there are no dynamic relations between the categories – after all, a category is defined in terms of the features of a species that are distinctive. Most psychiatric textbooks, from Emil Kraepelin's *Lehrbuch* to its legitimate contemporary heir the American Psychiatric Association's *Diagnostic and Statistical Manual of Mental Disorders*, consider patients, at least in principle, to belong to one particular pathology with distinctive features (symptoms), without the possibility of any dynamic relation between these pathologies. Things are, at least potentially, completely different with Freud. Since the different psychopathologies reveal universal human tendencies, they can (and should) in principle also be considered in dynamic relation to one another. Freud does not develop this insight in great detail, but his famous saying that neurosis is the negative of perversion is a perfect illustration of such a dynamic and internal relation.

Sexuality and/as pleasure

What, then, is sexuality when its model is hysteria? What aspects of human existence can be highlighted via the study of hysteria? To answer such questions, Freud first relates hysteria to the perversions by arguing that hysterical symptoms are nothing but the converted expressions of the drives that can be described as "perverse" by nature. Based on his analysis of the sexual objects and aims, which dismisses a functional interpretation of the drives, Freud deduces that the sexual drive consists of an amalgam of components manifesting itself in a variety of "perverse" objects and aims. It is the non-functional, non-normative interpretation of sexuality that makes it possible to name the "normal" sexual drive "perverse," and it is the study of hysteria that substantiates this claim. Hysteria highlights the same psychic processes and mechanisms that we find in normal human existence, and the hysteric symptoms are expressions of the perverse nature of the sexual drive. Freud's dictum that neurosis is the negative of perversion can thus be read as follows: perversion is "positive" in the sense that the term *perverse* describes, first, the nature of the sexual drives and, second, the direct and concrete manifestation of these drives in phantasy or acts; the psychoneuroses result from the excessive degree of repression of the sexual drives (Freud 1905a: 25). We can thus witness in hysteria the manifestation of the perverse nature of sexuality; that is, the so-called aberrations we recognize as variations of so-called normal sexuality.[18]

According to Freud, the hysterical constitution highlights three central aspects of sexuality (Haute & Geyskens 2012). First, there is the bisexual disposition. Freud credits Wilhelm Fliess for his innovative work on this issue (Freud 1905a: 27, 71). Indeed, bisexuality had long been a topic of Fliess's biological theories, but it was Freud's own clinical findings in the study of hysteria that had shown that (non-anatomical) bisexuality is constitutive of hysteria. Notably, the Dora case further substantiated the hysteric's random switching between male and female roles and male and female objects. A few years earlier, Freud had already concluded from this that there were always four individuals involved in every sexual act: the male/female subject orientation and the male/female object (Freud 1985: 364). In spite of this, and of the fact that he originally intended to give his text on the theory of sexuality the title *Die menschliche Bisexualität* (Ibid.: 448), Freud does not provide a comprehensive theory of bisexuality in *Three Essays*. The second aspect of sexuality entails the "tendencies to every kind of anatomical extension of sexual activity," which one finds in hysteria more often and more intensely in comparison with normal sexuality (Freud 1905a: 27). Freud is referring here to another observation from his clinical experience with hysterical patients: their symptom formations always pointed to an inclination toward the oral or anal erogenous zones that produced pleasure – that is, sexual excitation – in early childhood and were then repressed through disgust and shame. These inclinations registered that the (partial) sexual drives – oral and anal drives but also perverse opposite tendencies, such as exhibitionism and voyeurism – were still exerting pressure, though they now produced only unpleasure. Eating disorders or feelings of suffocation, for instance,[19] were the typical symptoms that could be traced back to oral sexual pleasure and disgust (Ibid.: 27, 43). Third, and relatedly, Freud developed the idea that human sexuality has to overcome its initial mixing with excremental functions. In *Three Essays*, Freud only mentions this idea in passing (Ibid.: 15), but he develops it in much greater detail in his text on Dora. Here he writes: "[t]he Early Christian Fathers' '*inter urinas et faeces nascimur*' clings to sexual life and cannot be detached from it in spite of every effort at idealization" (Freud 1905d: 31).[20] The separation of sexuality from the excremental functions, according to Freud, can only be realized through the introduction of the typically human affects of disgust and shame (and guilt) and through a complex process of idealization. More specifically, the hysterical problematic is characterized by the imminent and insurmountable threat of a contamination of the sexual by the excremental (Haute 2018).

These three aspects of the hysterical constitution confirm what Freud had already hinted at: what we call the sexual drive is actually a composition or bundle of partial drives (Freud 1905a: 29). In the 1915 edition of *Three Essays*, Freud will insert a passage on the theory of the drives summarizing a few basic notions from "Instincts and Their Vicissitudes" (also published in 1915). In that passage, he will argue that the sexual partial drives in fact originate from one of the two forms of excitation of the organs. Freud is referring here to what he calls the two primal drives – namely, the drives of self-preservation (ego drives) and the sexual drive – which are first aimed at organ pleasure before entering the service of the reproduction function. It is only then that the sexual drive becomes recognizable as such and reveals its actual purpose and content: the production of new individuals (Freud 1905c: 67–68, 1915: 124–126). With the appearance in 1915 of this strong version of the drive dichotomy, a functional approach enters the text, linking Freud's new interpretation of the primal drives to the body of thought he had so explicitly dismissed in 1905 as an inaccurate fable.

But what does Freud tell us in 1905? When discussing the partial drives he writes that they are susceptible to further analysis. He then writes a few sentences that were deleted from the 1915 edition and all subsequent editions:

> In addition to a "drive," which is not itself sexual and which has its source in motor impulses, we can discern in the partial drives a contribution from an organ receiving stimuli (e.g., the skin, the mucous membrane, or a sense organ). An organ of this kind will be described in this connection as an "erogenous zone" – as being the organ whose excitation lends the drive a sexual character.
>
> *(Freud 1905a: 29)*[21]

The passage can be read in (at least) two ways. The first reading would argue that there is *one* primal drive that may become sexual through the erogenous zones.

The idea would then be that Freud proposes one primal drive that is differentiated into various domains and functions, of which the sexual function is one. The second reading of the passage would argue that there is *some* impulse that we can first identify as a sexual drive through its link with the erogenous zones. In 1905, while distancing himself from the perspective of his predecessors who gave a strictly functional interpretation of the genital/sexual instinct (preservation of the species), Freud was still uncertain about the exact nature and status of the drives.[22] But this did not prevent him from maintaining the Darwinian idea that psychic life is characterized by two – and only two[23] – fundamental tendencies: sexuality and self-preservation (drive for food intake). In the famous passage on sensual sucking (discussed later), Freud distinguishes between sexual pleasure and satisfaction on the one hand and the need for taking nourishment on the other. He does not speak here of a nutrition drive (or instinct for self-preservation), but he does distinguish between the sexual and the nonsexual, associating the latter with hunger and the need for nutrition. Since sensual sucking seems completely independent of the need for nutrition, according to Freud, we have no choice but to consider it sexual.

The excitation of bodily zones, such as the skin or mucous membranes, determines the sexual character of the drive. The question now arises as to what Freud means by "sexual" when it is defined relative to the excitation of zones and organs. In the second essay, Freud addresses the question of the origin and nature of sexuality in a section on the autoerotic manifestations of infantile sexuality. The starting point and model for his discussion of these manifestations is the phenomenon of sensual sucking (*Lutschen* or *Wonnesaugen*), a rhythmic oral activity (often combined with tugging some sensitive part of the body) that he describes as a sexual activity. Why and in what sense is sensual sucking sexual? Freud observes that sensual sucking "absorbs all attention, making the child either fall asleep or experience a motor reaction in a kind of orgasm" (Ibid.: 41; Geyskens 2005: 21–28; Westerink 2018). This hardly seems to answer our question. Freud's main argument is that this pleasure is sexual because it is essentially autoerotic and non-functional.[24] It has nothing to do with food intake and hence is not related to self-preservation – the need for food or the satisfaction of hunger. Freud here mainly applies his basic Darwinian scheme that whatever is not related to self-preservation is *for that very reason* sexual.[25]

It was Havelock Ellis who first coined the term *autoerotism*. He described it as "a spontaneous sexual emotion generated in the absence of an external stimulus proceeding, directly or indirectly, from another person" (Ellis 1900: 161ff). The typical forms of autoerotism, found almost exclusively in puberty and adult life, were sexual orgasm during sleep, erotic daydreams, and masturbation as well as the experience of sexual stimulation through the vibratory motion of machines and vehicles. According to Ellis, these autoerotic manifestations were mostly accompanied by sexual phantasies about other, absent persons. Freud moves beyond Ellis's conception of autoerotism when he uses it to describe the infantile experience of sexual pleasure; moreover, he defines autoerotism more radically than Ellis as being strictly without object. For Freud, autoerotism as we find it in early infancy is not about sexual phantasies since phantasy always implies an object (as discussed later).[26]

It is nothing but a physical-pleasurable activity originating from the "drive" and the excitability of erogenous zones. Nevertheless, Freud says that there is a primal activity that triggers sensual sucking, and this activity is breast-sucking. At first glance, it might appear as if sensual sucking therefore depends on the presence or absence of an object, but strictly speaking, this is not the case. The breast, or one of its surrogates, such as a milk bottle, is only a thing by means of which the infant discovers that sucking is pleasurable.[27] More concretely, while sucking at the mother's breast, the lips of the infant behave as an erogenous zone, and the warm milk creates a pleasurable excitation that the infant will later try to reproduce (Freud 1905a: 42). In other words, this is what Freud in the third essay will describe as "fore-pleasure" (Ibid.: 64); that is, *pleasure as the excitation of erogenous zones*, which should be distinguished from pleasure in terms of a release of tension (pleasure as absence of unpleasure). This implies that the infant's relation to the breast – or attachment to the object providing the milk – is not essential to sexuality. Freud's reference to Moll's theory of sexuality in this context is telling: infantile sexuality (sexual pleasure) cannot be reduced to biological functions (detumescence drive) or to loving attachment (contrectation drive). Breasts or bottles are mere instruments in the discovery of autoerotic pleasure. The objects of sensual sucking and tugging are not substitute objects for a supposedly absent first object, as is often argued (e.g., Lacan 1966; Quindeau 2014: 40). The child discovers that its own organs and body parts can be used to produce pleasure, and this *use* of body parts is to be distinguished from either the present function (e.g., food intake) or the later function (e.g., reproduction) of specific organs and body parts. The paradigm for this infantile sexuality, Freud writes, is *the lips kissing themselves* (Freud 1905a: 43).

Nonetheless, Freud is not as clear on this topic as it would at first seem. Further on in the text, when Freud discusses the transformations of puberty, he writes that while sexual satisfaction was still linked to ingestion, the sexual drive had a sexual object outside of the body – namely, the mother's breast – and it is for this reason, Freud adds, that breast-sucking is the model for all later object relations, and, conversely, every later "finding of an object" (*Objektfindung*) is nothing but "a re-finding of it" (*Wiederfindung*) (Ibid.: 73). This statement only seemingly contradicts what we said about the autoerotic character of infantile sexuality.[28] We know already that it is not so much the breast itself but rather the warm milk that creates the pleasurable excitation the child is actively seeking. More generally, sexuality gets directed toward an object as such only at the beginning of puberty. Only from puberty onward is pleasure sought in relation to the object that can provide it. Once this is the case, the erogenous zones are reinvested from the perspective of adult object-related sexuality. The breast can now acquire a meaning that it could not have had before. Hence, it is only retrospectively, in puberty, that breast-sucking attains paradigmatic value.

The idea that finding the object is inevitably re-finding it has been very influential in the history of psychoanalytic thinking. In particular, the idea of an irreducible distance or difference between the object we find and the object we have lost has been used to defend the idea that the drive and desire in Freud originate in negativity and that it is precisely this structural difference that would be the motor of psychic life.[29] According to Freud, however, what we lost is not so much an object but a specific regime of autoerotic pleasure. More importantly, Freud does not deduce from this state of affairs that negativity plays a central role in psychic life. On the contrary, the drive is a force that literally drives the human being forward and that seeks a release of tension. In Freud, therefore, the drive should not be understood as negativity.

One should not deduce from the fact that infantile sexuality is essentially autoerotic and should be described in physiological terms that phantasies do not play an essential role in pathogenesis. In "My Views on the Part Played by Sexuality in the Aetiology of the Neuroses," Freud writes that in the years prior to the publication of *Three Essays*, he became progressively aware not only of the importance of a sexual constitution and of hereditary factors but also of the role phantasies play in the creation of neurotic symptoms (Freud 1906). Freud's text on the Dora case, which was published in the same year as *Three Essays* and which serves as its clinical counterpart, can help us to better understand Freud's thinking here. Indeed, in this text Freud links Dora's symptomatic cough to a phantasy of fellatio that she finds repulsive and therefore represses. However, Freud is very clear about the fact that this phantasy is created during puberty. Mr. K's declaration of his love for Dora during a trip to the lake when she is sixteen years old reminds her of an earlier seduction by the same Mr. K. On the previous occasion, he had tried to embrace and kiss her in his grocery shop, and in that moment she felt his erect penis against her body. The unpleasurable affect that accompanies this feeling is displaced: "Dora was overcome by the unpleasurable feeling that is proper to the tract of the mucous membrane at the entrance of the alimentary canal – that is by disgust" (Freud 1905d: 29). Freud links this displacement from the genital to the oral zone to the fact that as a child Dora was an enthusiastic sensual sucker and that this disposed the oral zone to playing a crucial role in her adult life. In Dora's sexuality the oral zone (and its repression) plays a predominant role (Ibid.: 30). The displacement of the affective rejection of Mr. K's aggressive advances from the genital to the oral zone clearly testifies to this. It also illustrates what Freud means when he writes that the erogenous zones are identical to the hysterogenic zones and that they show the same characteristics (Freud 1905a: 44–45).

It is this first scene and the unpleasant affect that goes along with it that is reactivated through Mr. K's declaration of love at the lake. At the moment of the first trauma, Dora had not yet entered puberty and for that reason could not link this event to concrete sexual representations, but now she is in puberty and knows that parts of the body other than the genitals can be used for sexual gratification and sexual intercourse (Freud 1905d: 47). At that stage of her life, Dora was very preoccupied with the relationship between her father and Frau K, and she actively participated in it in many ways. It comes as no surprise, then, "that with her spasmodic cough, which, as is usual, was referred for its exciting stimulus to a tickling in her throat, she pictured to herself a scene of sexual gratification *per os* between the two people whose love-affair occupied her mind so incessantly" (Ibid.: 48). It is this phantasy that is expressed in the spasmodic cough, which is one of Dora's most characteristic symptoms. Once again, we see that it is only at the beginning of puberty that sexuality receives an object and becomes phantasmatic; hence, only from puberty onward will phantasies play a role in pathogenesis.

We recognize here the structure of "deferred action" (*Nachträglichkeit*) that Freud had developed earlier in his work, and more particularly in "Project for a Scientific Psychology" in 1895 and *The Interpretation of Dreams* in 1900.[30] This deferred action cannot be understood apart from the crucial role puberty plays in the development of the human being.[31] In his "Project," for instance, Freud explains how Emma is seduced by a shopkeeper who touches her genitals through her clothing (Freud 1985: 354–356). At first, this event remains without real consequences, Freud continues, because at that time Emma is not yet capable of understanding the sexual nature of the shopkeeper's advances. It is only at a later time – at the beginning of puberty – that things change dramatically. When Emma enters a clothing shop, the original scene threatens to become conscious again. But Emma is in puberty now and immediately grasps the sexual meaning of the original scene. She runs away in terror and develops a phobia for this type of shop. Of course, in 1895 Freud does not yet have a concept of infantile sexuality, but we already find here the idea that a first event receives a completely new meaning when it is remembered in a second moment after puberty has begun.[32]

Drive and instinct

Thus far we have not addressed the question of how Freud's concept of the drive relates to that of instinct. Based on the fact that Freud does not mention the word "instinct" (*Instinkt*) in *Three Essays*, one might be tempted to conclude that Freud's 1905 views of the drive are a radical dismissal of the theories held by predecessors like Krafft-Ebing, for whom drive and instinct appear to be synonymous concepts. For Moll, for example, instinct and drive indicate the objective and subjective dimension of the same process: the natural instinct for reproduction is subjectively manifested and experienced in a drive for coitus with a heterosexual adult partner.[33] But does the absence of the concept of instinct indeed point at a radical critique of his predecessors' use of the concepts instinct and drive? Does Freud's concept of drive stand in opposition to a concept of instinct that indicates the physiological and psychological orientation toward predetermined objects and aims?

From the first sentence of *Three Essays* we can already conclude that things are more complicated. Freud writes: "[t]he fact of genital needs in man and animal is expressed in biology by the assumption of a genital drive. This drive is considered analogous to the desire for food, that is, to hunger" (Freud 1905a: 1). From this statement, it follows that the concept of drive is used to describe needs and driving forces found in both human and animal life. Freud here in no way suggests a fundamental difference between human drives and animal instincts. Notably, also in the third essay – "The Transformations of Puberty" – any distinction between human drive and animal instinct is relativized when Freud introduces a heteronormative perspective on the normal and natural sexual life of adolescents and adults. He writes:

> [w]ith the arrival of puberty, changes set in that are supposed to lead infantile sexual life to its final, normal shape. . . . Now there is a new sexual aim. . . . The normality of sex life is warranted solely by an exact convergence of the two currents directed toward the sexual object and the sexual aim. It is like the breakthrough of a tunnel driven through from both directions.
>
> *(Ibid.: 61)*

In this passage Freud undermines his critique of the "poetic fable" when adopting a functional and teleological perspective on adult sexuality similar to the views held by Krafft-Ebing, Moll, and others. In this context, Freud also reasons that the transformation of sexuality in puberty must be understood in terms of being grounded in and originating from physiological processes and not as originating, for example, from individual preferences or cultural norms; the section on chemical theory gives evidence of this (Ibid.: 69–70). It seems that Freud returns to a theory in which adolescent and adult sexuality can be understood in terms of biological processes and functions aimed at reproduction, as if the theory of infantile sexuality were needed only to develop ideas on the period Freud's predecessors found hard to understand: the infantile "premature" period in which the sexual organs are not prepared to fulfill their natural task.

Apparently, Freud's concept of drive in the third essay seems to have a number of "instinctive" characteristics. In sum, *Three Essays* does not provide a theory of sexuality based on a sharp distinction between drive (in human life – in culture) and instinct (in animal life – in nature).[34] From the absence of the word *Instinkt* in *Three Essays*, we should therefore not conclude that Freud radically distances himself from the conceptual framework of his predecessors; to the contrary, we instead see that for him the question of the distinction between drive and instinct is not a pressing problem.

Another – in our view a more fundamental – distinction comes to the fore in *Three Essays*. Although neither explicitly stated as such nor systematically applied, Freud differentiates between sexual drive (*Sexualtrieb*) and genital drive (*Geschlechtstrieb*), associating the first predominantly with infantile sexuality and referring to the second always either in the context of a critique of the "poetic fable" or in his elaborations on pubertal and adult sexuality.[35] The concepts of sexual drive and genital drive thus refer to two sexual "regimes": infantile sexuality, which is autoerotic, polymorphous perverse, and without an object, and adult sexuality, which is organized around the primacy of the genitals and functionally aimed at reproduction with a heterosexual partner.

Seduction, trauma, and disposition

The Dora case allows us to examine another point of great importance for properly understanding the first edition of *Three Essays*. In the beginning of his account,

Freud states that the psychic conditions for hysteria that he and Josef Breuer had described in their *Studies on Hysteria* – psychic trauma, conflict between the affects, and a disturbance in the sphere of sexuality – are also present in the Dora case (Freud 1905d: 24). This statement seems to contradict the most classical historiographical interpretation of Freudian thinking. This historiography wants us to believe that in 1897 Freud gave up his seduction theory of psychopathology in general and hysteria in particular – "I no longer believe in my neurotica" (Freud 1985: 264) – and that henceforth he understood the traumatic stories of his patients as distorted expressions of oedipal phantasies.[36] But how, then, can we explain the complete absence of references to the Oedipus complex in both the Dora case and the first edition of *Three Essays*?[37] All references to this complex were introduced in later editions, especially in the footnotes to the edition of 1920. It is clear that there are very good reasons to closely examine the passages in *Three Essays* where Freud is speaking of trauma and seduction and their relation to the neuroses. Freud summarizes the evolution of his views on the etiological significance of sexual traumata for neuroses as follows:

> I cannot admit that I overestimated its frequency or significance in my 1896 paper on "The Aetiology of Hysteria," though I did not then know that persons who remained normal might have had the same experiences in their childhood, and therefore placed more emphasis on the significance of seduction than on the factors of sexual constitution and development.
>
> *(Freud 1905a: 50)*

He further adds, "[O]bviously seduction is not required for the awakening of the child's sexual life; such awakening can also come about spontaneously as a result of internal causes" (Ibid.). Freud's disbelief in his "neurotica" did not mean that he would henceforth think that the traumata about which patients told him were imaginings in need of an (oedipal?) explanation; nor did it mean that he would refuse to accept the frequent occurrence of sexual seduction between adults and children (or between children). The statement that he did not overestimate the frequency of seduction in "The Aetiology of Hysteria" (Freud 1896b) also relativizes the idea that Freud gave up his traumatic theory of neurosis because he could not admit that there were as many perverted adults and fathers as his theory presupposed (Masson 1984). Things clearly are much more complex than is sometimes admitted (Davidson 1984).[38]

The term *neurotica* is a substantivized adjective in the nominative plural of the neuter gender (or, to be more precise, the accusative plural, in Freud's original formulation of this statement) and refers to Freud's "theory of the neuroses." Freud here addresses his theory of the traumatic origin of psychopathology. It is this theory, and not the traumatic stories of his patients, that he no longer believes. In other words, Freud questions the etiological significance of traumata and not their truth value. Indeed, *Three Essays* thematizes the disposition at the basis of hysteria. It explains how the hereditary or acquired exaggeration of some of the characteristics of this disposition leads to the development of hysterical symptoms. Seduction is traumatic for Freud because it confronts the child with a sexual object at a time when it is physiologically not yet ready for it. In other words, seduction does not respect the autoerotic character of infantile sexuality. This explains why sexual traumata can have all kinds of devastating effects. But Freud no longer considers these traumata to be a necessary cause for the genesis of hysterical pathology; nor do they constitute sufficient causes in most cases. Consider once again the Dora case: Dora's history is structured around two traumatic events. At no point does Freud question the truth value of these two events. He just takes them for granted. However, these events alone cannot explain Dora's hysteria. Quite the contrary, they become extremely meaningful and acquire a traumatic character only because of Dora's hysterical disposition.[39] Hence, according to Freud, Dora's reaction when Mr. K embraced her in his grocery shop also testifies to "the contradictory enigma of hysteria through identifying the pair of opposites [characteristic of hysteria] of a sexual rejection taken too far on the one hand, and an excessively felt sexual need, on the other" (Ibid.: 25). Aversion itself is linked to the contamination of the sexual with the excremental that we discussed earlier (Freud 1905d: 31). Dora's traumata are not the cause of her hysteria, but rather are the occasion that allows her hysterical disposition to be activated and expressed. There is nothing strange, then, about Freud's claim that his understanding of Dora's pathology is an extension of his earlier work on hysteria and, more particularly, of his *Studies in Hysteria*. Indeed, in his study on Dora and in *Three Essays*, Freud recalibrates the meaning and importance of sexual traumata in relation to a universal sexual disposition, but he at no point repudiates their reality or denies their possible noxious effects.

Oedipal relations and the incest barrier

At no point in the first edition of *Three Essays* does Freud take the infantile Oedipus complex as a possible explanation for psychopathology. Instead, as we have seen, he defends an organic or dispositional theory of neurosis in which trauma still plays a significant role. The absence of any reference to the Oedipus complex is not simply a matter of fact.[40] At this point in Freud's intellectual development, an infantile Oedipus complex is a theoretical impossibility. The Oedipus complex primarily consists of the positive and negative sexual ties toward the child's parents. It therefore presupposes that infantile sexuality has become objectal and is no longer strictly autoerotic – a transformation that does not happen until the beginning of puberty.[41] It follows that the oedipal themes that we find in culture and that Freud discovers in the stories of his patients are characteristic of puberty. The parents are likely to be the first (phantasmatic) objects of the libido, but the investment in these objects occurs at a moment after the latency period, when the incest barrier has been put in place (Freud 1905a: 75–77). Freud states that in contradistinction to the reaction formations, the incest barrier is a cultural demand of society that forces young people to direct their sexual interests outside of the family to help establish higher social units.[42]

But how, then, are we to understand the references to Oedipus in Freud's earlier work? In *The Interpretation of Dreams* and *Fragment of an Analysis of a Case of Hysteria*, he calls the Oedipus legend a poetical elaboration of the typical relation of children to their parents (Freud 1900: 257ff, 1905d: 56). We can still be moved by Sophocles's tragedy because it reminds us of an important aspect of our own childhood relation with our parents. But this does not imply that in these early texts Freud understands the neuroses from the perspective of a psychological Oedipus complex that would explain their nuclear structure. In the study on Dora, for instance, he explicitly writes that Dora's infantile relation to her father is summoned up in puberty to protect her from her love for Mr. K. An old love is reactivated to protect her from a current love. One can hardly call this interpretation oedipal in the classical sense of the word since such an interpretation would understand the actual love for Mr. K as a disguised repetition of the old (oedipal) one for the father and not the other way around (Blass 1992; Haute & Geyskens 2012: 54–56). In Freud's early work, King Oedipus can more plausibly be seen to function as an "archetype" for the modern (neurotic) subject. The figure of King Oedipus has an emblematic value for our tragic destiny (Roudinesco 2014).[43] But this reference is still far removed from the idea of a psychological complex that structures the development of the human psyche in the infantile period and that regulates our progressive inscription in the world of culture. It is only when Freud gives up the strict dichotomy between infantile (autoerotic) sexuality and pubertal objectal sexuality in the years following his study on infantile sexual researches and theories (Freud 1908a) and the case study of Little Hans and the boy's first sexual object choices (Freud 1909a) that such a psychological complex and its place in the developmental process becomes theoretically conceivable.[44] Similarly, it is only when the genesis and status of the object become an explicit problematic issue for Freud that the Oedipus complex can and will acquire a structural role in the development of the psyche.[45]

The problem of object relations

All of this does not prevent Freud from remaining quite ambiguous when describing the status of objects and object relations in early infancy (Blass 2017). He writes that even at the moment when sexual activity proper separates from ingestion and becomes autoerotic, an important part of the sexual relations remains present in the relation with the persons who take care of the vital needs of the infant:

> [t]hroughout the entire period of latency, the child learns to love other people who help it in its helplessness and satisfy its needs – a love on the model and in continuation of the relationship of the infant to its nursing caregivers.
>
> *(Freud 1905a: 73)*

Freud is speaking here about the tender feelings (*Zärtlichkeit*) of the child for its caregivers. The problem we are confronted with is a familiar one: since Freud mentions only two fundamental tendencies that govern the human psyche – a sexual drive and the need for nutrition (drive for food intake) – all relations to the surrounding world have to be explained in terms of either one or the other. Nevertheless, it is very hard to situate tenderness within this dichotomy: it cannot be reduced to the vital needs of hunger and thirst, nor is it merely sexual. Freud solves this problem by linking tenderness to inhibited sexuality. Tenderness is essentially a mode of sexuality. It is sexuality that is inhibited with regard to its aim ("attenuated libido") (Ibid.: 76). In other words, Freud explains all relations to objects (persons) in terms of libidinal ties, not in terms of self-preservation.

What is missing here is a theory of social instinct or "attachment" that would have allowed Freud not only to give tenderness a status of its own that cannot be reduced to sexuality but also to understand it as an original and fundamental dimension of human existence that does not require an explanation in terms of a specific individual's life (such as the experience of being cared for). Darwin had already pointed toward this in his 1871 *The Descent of Man* when arguing for a social instinct that becomes manifest in social bonds of love or sympathy, notably when in the course of evolution this instinct is strengthened by parental and filial affections (such as in the case of human beings) (Darwin 1981: 72ff). In this view, the attachment to objects does not result from a mere biological dependency (nutrition) on the presence of the mother but instead should be seen as originating from an inherited social instinct that is not specific to human nature. Already for Darwin it was clear that what we would now call attachment behavior was rooted in evolution.[46] It can be understood on evolutionary grounds and in terms of evolutionary benefits. In other words, it is a primary drive that belongs to our very nature and does not need an explanation at the level of the individual (Bowlby 1969: 210–234). Would it not be rather remarkable that the explanation for a whole series of behaviors and feelings occurring in most mammals would have to be completely different for humans? Furthermore, children may also be attached to persons who are not at all occupied with the satisfaction of their needs (and who sometimes have the opposite aim). Whatever the case may be, Freud thinks that the sexual drive finds an object at the beginning of puberty by following the pathways that have been traced by tender relationships toward the caregivers, primarily the parents. He writes: "[c]ertainly the most natural thing for the child to do would be to choose as sexual objects the very persons whom it has loved since childhood with what may be called attenuated libido" (Freud 1905a: 75–76).

It is not only the distinction between food intake and sexual drives that causes problems for Freud, or that at least needs to be put in perspective. Freud links the partial drives to the different erogenous zones that he discovered through the study of the perversions. He takes the oral drive as a paradigm for the study of these zones.[47] This allows him to characterize infantile sexuality as essentially autoerotic, "without an object," and non-phantasmatic. But having linked the traumatic character of seduction to the fact that it introduces an object to the sexual drive at a moment when the young child is not physiologically ready for it, Freud must admit that infantile sexuality entails components that are from the outset directed toward an external object.[48] Such components are the drives for watching and cruelty. At the same time, Freud is far from clear about the exact nature of these components. He writes, for instance, that despite its close link to sexuality, the drive for watching is initially independent of it. But this statement is followed immediately by another one in which Freud says not only that seduction can "sexualize" – or, more precisely, "pervert" – the drive for watching from early on in life but also that this sexualization – the pressing need to see other people's genitalia, for instance – can occur as a spontaneous expression of infantile sexuality (Ibid.: 52). We find the same uncertainty with regard to the cruelty component of the sexual drive. Freud states that the cruel impulses find their origin in sources independent from sexuality but which from very early on become linked to it through anastomosis (Ibid.). With regard to these uncertainties, we could accuse Freud of inconsistency, or we could appreciate the fact that he does not lock himself into one model and that he tries, on the contrary, to do justice to the phenomena that seem to contradict his original insights. This surely brings some imbalance into the text, but at the same time it makes it possible to read it as the articulation of a problem or set of related problems, rather than as a set of answers that must be dogmatically accepted or rejected. Freud, remarkably enough, never tries to hide the problems that haunt his own system.[49]

It is worthwhile to examine one such moment in which Freud is confronted with the limits of his own paradigm. As discussed, according to Freud, infantile sexuality is nothing but an organic inscription on the body (autoerotism). There is nothing dramatic about infantile sexuality. Freud compares it to tickles that one can experience in different parts of the body (the erogenous zones). But is this a tenable position? We also already know that the object – the breast, for example – does not play a significant role in this context. It can be instrumental in eliciting the excitement that the child wants to repeat, but at no point is it intended *as such* by the drives. Jean Laplanche famously calls such a view "ipsocentric" (Laplanche 1992: 57). This approach implies that infantile sexuality develops out of itself from an autoerotic to an objectal stage. The other plays no structural role in this development, except as a catalyst: she or he has no determining significance for the development that she or he sets in motion. But elsewhere in his text, Freud introduces a new figure. It is no longer the breast/milk that causes pleasure in spite of itself, but rather the mother who takes the child as "full-fledged sexual object." Freud writes:

> [a] child's contact with its caregiver affords it an unending source of sexual excitation and satisfaction emanating from its erogenous zones. This is especially so since the caregiver – the mother, as a rule – herself bestows upon the child feelings derived from her own sexual life: she strokes it, kisses it, rocks it, and quite clearly treats it as a substitute for a full-fledged sexual object. *(Freud 1905a: 74)*

Freud interprets this state of affairs from his own ipsocentric and physiological perspective. He does not give any special weight or importance to the mother's sexuality, which seems clearly implied here. Instead, he again immediately reduces the role of the mother to awakening the child's sexuality through her tender activities. These activities, he adds, prepare the future intensity of the sexual drive:

> [s]he is only fulfilling her duty in teaching the child to love. After all, the child is meant to grow into a competent person with vigorous sexual needs, and to accomplish in life all the things that human beings are impelled to do by their drives.
>
> *(Ibid.)*[50]

Everything here is a matter of the right measure. We cannot do without a sufficient amount of tenderness, but too much tenderness – and excitation – prevents the child from learning that, in matters of love, one cannot always have what one wants. Thus, Freud's argumentation first equates taking the child as a "full-fledged sexual object" with tenderness, and then reduces the significance of tender feelings to the eliciting of the right amount of pleasurable (sexual) excitation. But is not initiating a tender, caring relationship with a child quite different from taking it as a "full-fledged sexual object"? It is especially difficult to reconcile Freud's exclusively "physiological" reasoning with his statement that the mother as a rule bestows upon the child feelings derived from her own sexual life and quite clearly treats it as a substitute for a full-fledged sexual object. We have already mentioned the problematic status of tenderness in Freud's text, but here things become even more complex: if the tender and caring relation with the child is essentially contaminated by adult sexual phantasies – and what else could taking the child as a "full-fledged sexual object" mean? – is it still possible to describe the effects of this relation in purely physiological terms? Does this contamination not imply that the child is confronted with the sexual (phantasmatic) life of the adult (and not just with a surplus of excitation) at a moment when it is not yet ready for it, and that this exceeds its capacities? Jean Laplanche systematized this problematic under the heading of a "generalized seduction" (Laplanche 1987; Haute & Geyskens 2004: 103–144; Quindeau 2014: 24–28). The adult unknowingly and unwillingly confronts the child with sexual messages to which it has to respond without having at its disposal the proper means – intellectual, affective, or cognitive – to understand them. Hence, the efforts of translation the child is forced to make are structurally incomplete. They inevitably leave a remainder that Laplanche identifies with the sexual unconscious. In Freud, infantile sexuality has nothing to do with the cognitive or emotional understanding (or lack thereof) of the other's or one's own motives, intentions, or phantasies. Freud thinks about infantile sexuality in purely physiological terms. Nevertheless, in his text we find elements – the seductive mother, the ambiguous status of the drive for watching – that indicate the limits of his model and that might lead us to thematize (infantile) sexuality in another manner.

Freud himself will explicitly do this from 1910 onward. In his 1910 *Five Lectures on Psycho-Analysis*, he writes that his focus on the somatic aspects of infantile sexuality had led him to pay less attention to the psychic effects of the child's helplessness and need of care. He argues that the parents' tender feelings and the child's responses to these feelings are always accompanied by "elements of sexual excitation." This results in the child taking "both of its parents, and more particular one of them, as the object of erotic wishes" (Freud 1910a: 47). The child thus responds to an initiative taken by the parents.[51] It is this constellation that now and for the first time Freud will identify as the oedipal "nuclear complex of every neurosis," i.e., the Oedipus complex. In other words, whereas in the 1905 *Three Essays* Freud had articulated the child's sexual pleasure and excitation in terms of autoerotic activities, in 1910 he shifts attention toward the child's first object choices as a source of sexual excitation and erotic wishes.[52]

Puberty and the organization of pleasure

Let us return once more to the text of *Three Essays*, specifically to the third essay, "The Transformations of Puberty." In the first edition of the text, Freud hardly mentions the developmental perspective that is so characteristic of both his own later works and most psychoanalytic theory. In 1905, Freud distinguishes only two developmental "phases": infantile masturbation and its return at the age of three or four years. All emphasis is on the structural changes that occur at the beginning of puberty. We are already familiar with some of these structural changes. In general, the beginning of puberty marks the moment when "the erogenous zones become subordinated to the primacy of the genital zone" (Freud 1905a: 61). During the infantile period, the genital zone functions like any other erogenous zone. In this period, the different partial drives seek pleasure independently of one another. It is only at the beginning of puberty that the genital zone becomes predominant. Freud is unclear about how we should understand this change and how it comes about. It primarily means that orgasmic pleasure – Freud calls it "end-pleasure" – can bring a halt to the preliminary pleasures we experience at the different erogenous zones. What does this mean?

We should remember that the link between the drive and its objects is essentially contingent. The reference to "fore-pleasure" and "end-pleasure" in a certain sense strengthens this sense of contingency (Ibid.: 64–65). As long as the difference between the genital zone and the other erogenous zones is exclusively thematized as a difference between two types of *pleasure*, Freud is not obliged to postulate an essential relation between the drive and a *specific* type of object. Both a homo- and a heterosexual object, for instance, can be involved in the production of "end-pleasure." From the perspective of pleasure, the nature of the object is irrelevant. This would be consistent with Freud's earlier statements on the status of the object, and it would have allowed him to continue the deconstruction of the relation between "normality" and pathology that he had begun in the two previous chapters of his text. Yet this is not what Freud does. On the contrary, he immediately links the notion of "end-pleasure," which belongs to the genital zone and genitality, to the idea of a heterosexual object choice.[53] Freud suddenly seems to think that, in principle, the possibility of "end-pleasure" goes together or should go together with the choice of a heterosexual object. Nothing in his text obliged him to give a privileged theoretical status to this choice. Indeed, his whole argumentation up to this point should have prevented him from doing so. In this way, Freud reintroduces the functionalist approach that characterized the psychiatric style of reasoning we discussed earlier.[54]

How do the different erogenous zones enter into the new structure that is dominated by the genital zone? According to Freud, they deliver the fore-pleasure that makes the orgasmic pleasure possible (Ibid.). More concretely, they orient the drive toward its fundamental aim: orgasm and (in the case of the male subject) the ejaculation that goes along with it.[55] Freud identifies pleasure fundamentally with a release of tension: an increase in tension is felt as unpleasure, and a release of tension is felt as pleasure. What characterizes the preliminary pleasures is that they are paradoxically accompanied by an increase in sexual tension. It is precisely this increase in tension – that in principle is felt as unpleasure – that compels us to continue until we reach the final outcome of this process: orgasm. Indeed, it is only orgasm that allows for a complete release of tension. The primacy that the genital zone attains in puberty relates not to the type of object that causes pleasure but to the fact that it allows for a different and more intense type of pleasure. The idea that in puberty pleasure is explicitly sought out in relation to an object – this is what differentiates infantile sexuality from adult (pubertal) sexuality – does not imply that this object should in principle be a heterosexual one. Such a claim contradicts the general outline of Freud's argument.

But things are even more complex. Not only is it unclear why the object of the genital drive should be a heterosexual one, but, following Freud's line of thinking, it is also unclear why we should give any privilege to the genital zone as such. Freud conceives the sexual drive in infancy as an amalgamation of components. The genital zone is one of these components but has no natural privilege. Affirming this privilege seems to reintroduce the identification of sexuality with the genital drive – even though it is this very identification Freud explicitly criticizes throughout *Three Essays*. And yet this identification is implied in the following passage that we find in the summary of Freud's text, which is meant to explain the origin of the perversions:

> [w]riters on the subject think, for instance, that the necessary precondition for a whole number of perverse fixations lies in an innate weakness of the sexual drive. In this form, this position seems to me untenable; it makes perfect sense, however, if what is meant is a constitutional weakness of one particular factor in the sexual drive, namely the genital zone – a zone which later takes over the function of combining the individual sexual activities for the purpose of reproduction. For if the genital zone is weak, this combination, which is required to take place at puberty, is bound to fail, and the strongest of the other components of sexuality will prevail in its activity as perversion.
>
> *(Ibid.: 86)*

Freud thus links the different perversions with a weakness of "one particular factor in the sexual drive, namely the genital zone." When the preliminary pleasures become too strong (and the genital zone, by contrast, too weak) and the accompanying tension is not strong enough, the sexual process can come to a standstill, which is exactly what happens in perversion. Arnold Davidson notes, for good reason, that this statement about the sexologists of Freud's day is quite astonishing. Freud criticizes them because they claim that the perversions are the effect of an innate weakness of the sexual drive and not of the genital component of this drive. But this is exactly what these sexologists always maintained and had to maintain in light of their interpretation of the sexual drive as a genital drive and its reproductive function. It is Freud who cannot say what he says given the argumentation he introduces in his text. The only thing Freud could have written while remaining consistent with his own thinking, Davidson concludes, is the following:

> [f]or if the genital zone is weak, this combination which often takes place at puberty (instead of: "in der Pubertät *geforderte* . . ."), will fail, and the strongest of the other components of sexuality will continue its activity (instead of: "wird ihre Betätigung *als Perversion durchsetzen*").
>
> *(Davidson 2001: 89)*

Freud struggles in this text not only with the limits of his own paradigm but also with the paradigm itself. There are clearly instances in which it looks as if Freud does not want to accept the consequences of his own reasoning.

There is yet another crucial element to highlight here. The subordination of the different erogenous zones to the genital zone changes the way in which they function. We had indicated that in puberty they are reinvested from the perspective of an essentially object-related adult sexuality. It is, as we know, only in this way that they can play a role in the sexual phantasies that are repressed in hysteria. But there is more at stake. Earlier, we discussed the idea that finding the object (in puberty) is essentially re-finding it, and in this context we stressed the paradoxical logic according to which *re*-finding implies a distance or a difference between what is found and what was initially lost. Something similar is at work with the pleasure we get from the different erogenous zones. To understand this, we have to look at the study on jokes Freud published in the same year as *Three Essays* as well as his study on Dora. Freud refers to this text when explaining the nature and functioning of preliminary pleasures.[56] What seems to interest him most here is the fact that we can laugh at our own jokes only through the laughter of the other.[57] It is only the laughter of the other that allows us to overcome the inhibitions that stand in the way of our pleasure. Freud seems to think that, in a similar way, we can find the autoerotic pleasures of our early childhood only through the use of the pleasure of the other. What does this mean?

The paradigm of infantile sexuality,[58] so we are told, is not the child at its mother's breast but the lips kissing themselves. The oral drive loses its force after some time; the infant stops sucking its own body parts even when not forced by adults to do so. The development of the genital zone at the beginning of puberty accompanies a renewed strengthening of the oral zone, which leads to a nervous tension that can be reduced by smoking and drinking or by hysterical vomiting. In these phenomena, the oral drive shows its new strength without giving any new pleasure. But some ferocious sensual suckers, says Freud, manage to become not only heavy smokers or drinkers but also "gourmets in kissing," with a tendency toward "perverse kissing." In this way, the old oral pleasures are brought to life again through the pleasure of the other, which is the new aim of sexual activity. Fore-pleasure is first and foremost pleasure at the pleasure of the other. Once again, we find an irrevocable distance between infantile sexuality and its reinvestment at the beginning of puberty.[59]

This logic of preliminary pleasure, together with the idea of infantile autoerotism being radically without object, determines Freud's theory of aesthetics: the asocial (non-objectal) pleasures of early childhood can be retrieved only through a social activity aimed at the pleasure of the other. In theater, for instance, we repeat the playful activity of children. However, the child's play is asocial; it is not essentially directed toward an audience (Freud 1908c: 421–422). Theater, on the contrary, is unthinkable apart from the audience for which it is performed.[60]

Deconstructing normativity

Freud's theory in the first version of *Three Essays* differs on many points from the image we have of his thinking and its genesis. This first version contains a radical deconstruction of the normative distinction between pathology and normality. But assuming for a moment that he had remained consistent with his own starting points, does this mean that Freud would have said that *in sexualibus* anything goes? We doubt it. Indeed, Freud explains why sexuality is intrinsically conflictual. The reaction formations he is talking about – in particular shame and disgust but also guilt and morality – imply that the experience of sexuality is never without inherent limitations. The need for variation also always involves potential conflict. In our opinion, this can also explain why sexuality is inevitably subject to (historical and contingent) law. Freud says not only that experiences of shame, guilt, disgust, and the like belong to the very nature of sexuality but also that the content of these experiences – *what* it is exactly that we consider to be disgusting or shameful – depends to a high degree on the social and cultural circumstances in which we live.[61] This implies that every culture is confronted with the inevitable task of providing concrete content to these experiences.[62] Or, in other words, no culture can escape from imposing concrete regulations on sexuality, but these regulations are not prescribed by nature. Culture is inscribed in already existing psychic patterns and dams and is thus not the "radical other" of nature. But this does not mean that nature can legitimize culture. What Freud wants to show is not so much that sexuality does not need regulation or legislation – perhaps the opposite – but that ultimately no such concrete regulation has a *fundamentum in re*. In this respect, Freud is essentially anti-Aristotelian.

Despite the critical potential of his theory, on several occasions Freud falls back into the "popular opinion" that he rejects. We have already discussed some of the passages that illustrate this tendency. These passages – such as the introductory paragraphs to "The Transformations of Puberty" – reintroduce a heteronormative perspective or reestablish a strict (and "natural") distinction between the normal and the pathological (in particular the perversions). Arnold Davidson correctly remarks that we should not interpret the tensions these passages introduce into the text as a deconstructive indeterminacy or an undecidability of the text. Rather, what is at stake is a certain mentality, a shared culture from which Freud could not escape. Davidson defines a mentality as "a set of mental habits or automatisms that characterize the collective understanding and representations of a population" (Davidson 2001: 91). Freud introduced a set of concepts that, at least in principle, enabled a rupture with the psychiatric style of reasoning that supported the mentality of his day – a mentality in which he also inevitably participated. Hence, it is the divergent temporality of the disappearance of an old mentality and the emergence of new concepts undermining it that can explain Freud's difficulty in grasping the radical character of his own thinking. The instability of his text seems to be a direct result of this state of affairs.

Disappearance of hysteria and reorganization of nosological categories

We have seen that in *Three Essays* hysteria provides the main model for the conceptualization of sexuality, and we have sketched the developments in Freud's writings until 1905 that led him to take hysteria as a model. Notably, the Dora case provided crucial insights into, for example, the importance of constitutional factors, erogenous zones, bisexuality, oral activity (sensual sucking), and disgust (Haute 2018; Westerink 2018). Seen from this perspective, we could say that *Three Essays* is his last major study in a sequence of studies of hysteria. Given the fact that Freud's clinical expertise and theoretical insights were largely built on his analyses of hysterical patients, and given the patho-analytic method Freud had already developed in earlier writings,[63] taking hysteria as a model for a theory of sexuality is consequently not that surprising. One might assume that Freud felt at least confident enough to approach sexuality from this perspective, viewing the status of hysteria as a clinical phenomenon and nosological category and the stability and significance of its characteristics and plausibility of his own insights as stable and consistent enough for the application of hysteria as model for a theory of sexuality. However, we have also seen that in the 1905 version of *Three Essays* several important unresolved questions and inconsistencies can be identified. It is in these moments that one recognizes the contestability and limitations of the model of hysteria.[64]

In later versions of *Three Essays*, Freud does not commit himself to strengthening the original paradigms. On the contrary, in the prefaces to the 1910 and 1915 editions he admits the work's "deficiencies and obscurities" and speaks of "[e]xpectations that cannot be fulfilled [because] a number of important problems of sexual life" are not properly dealt with in the text (Freud 1905c: 130). The newly inserted passages – especially the additions made to the 1915 and 1920 editions of the text – do not erase these deficiencies and problems but in fact further undermine his 1905 theory of sexuality and seem to lead Freud away from a number of his most radical intuitions found in the original edition. These new paragraphs sometimes bluntly contradict earlier ones that Freud nevertheless retains in the text. Henceforth, the instability of *Three Essays* we spoke of in the previous section is no longer a matter of a divergent temporality in which an old mentality persists alongside newly emerging concepts; rather, it is generated by an opposition between different theoretical models, approaches, and concepts. As we will discuss in detail in the next chapter, these new passages undermine some of the most crucial insights of the first edition. In other words, the inserted passages in the later editions do not support or complement the original model and theory but in fact undermine their plausibility and consistency. It is at this point that we must raise the question as to why the 1905 *Three Essays* would be Freud's last major text on hysteria.

Several scholars have drawn attention to the significance of shifts in the field of neurology and psychiatry around 1900 that also affected Freud's work. One of the main developments concerns the so-called disappearance of Charcotian hysteria; that is, the dramatic convulsive grand hysterical disorders as described in Charcot's writings of the 1870s and 1880s. This disappearance takes place at two levels. First, there is the fact that soon after the death of Charcot in 1893, the number of patients in the Salpêtrière in Paris suffering *la grande hystérie* rapidly declined. Second, there is the related fact that Charcot's successors – notably Joseph Babinski – strongly criticized the Charcotian concept and diagnosis of hysteria, arguing that hysteria, which Babinski now renamed pithiatism, was nothing but a transitory affliction making a person susceptible to autosuggestion. Hysterical paralyses, contractions, and other symptoms were in fact the results of organic diseases and defects and for this reason should not be called "hysterical." The Salpêtrian tradition officially came to an end at a meeting of Paris neurologists in 1908, when the full membership agreed to discard hysteria (Shorter 1992: 196–202; Micale 1993). The disappearance of Charcotian hysteria thus first of all took place in the context of developments in French neurology. These developments were already visible by the time Freud wrote his *Three Essays*, and even though he dealt with cases of *petite hystérie*, a problem emerged. How could a diagnostic category that seemed to have lost its relevance among practitioners and theoreticians of neurology remain the paradigm for understanding human sexuality and psychopathology? This problem became even more urgent when we consider the fact that not only was the status of hysteria fundamentally debated but so, too, were the other (neurological) categories – notably neurasthenia – with which Freud was most familiar.[65] The fields of neurology and psychiatry were rapidly changing, one innovation following the other. This not only concerned the disappearance, emergence, and reorganization of categories but also affected Freud's conceptual apparatus. His *Three Essays* gives evidence of this. He does not articulate his theory of sexuality within a strict neurological conceptual framework (neurons, impulses/stimuli [*Reize*], endogenous excitation, psychic energy, affect, discharge, etc.) as he did in the 1890s. Instead, the last major study of hysteria also marks the systematic introduction of the concept of drive into Freud's work – a concept that was already broadly accepted in sexological and psychiatric literature.

The disappearance of hysteria, however, is also limited; that is, it primarily concerns Charcot's *grande hystérie* in the French neurological literature. By contrast, hysteria remained an important concept in German psychiatric literature, which is evidenced by the major handbooks and textbooks by protagonists like Karl Jaspers, Emil Kraepelin, and Eugen Bleuler (Jaspers 1913: 168–169, 174–181; Kraepelin 1915: 1547–1706; Bleuler 1916: 378–397; Weber 2015). In this context, hysteria as a diagnosis and concept in its relation to other nosological categories was continued, reconsidered, and redefined. The limited, often dismissive, but sometimes also positive, reception of Freud's views on hysteria – particularly the idea of traumatic memories, the conversion of psychic conflicts, the cathartic method, and other aspects – in German psychiatric literature contributed to this. When psychiatrists during and after World War I were confronted with the phenomenon of shell shock in a male population, the category of hysteria could again provide service and gain weight in discussions. Shell shock was often interpreted in terms of traumatic neurosis, war neurosis, or war hysteria (*Kriegshysterie*),[66] with the focus placed not only on autosuggestion or physiological damage but also on psychogenic factors[67] such as "the flight into illness" and neurotic repression (Freud 1919a; Lerner 2003; Scull 2009: 153–173). In Freud's own writings, this trend is given evidence in his 1920 *Beyond the Pleasure Principle*. He writes that the traumatic neuroses one finds in shell shock patients do indeed share strong similarities with hysteria (Freud 1920: 12). He refers to his past studies on traumatic hysteria as "suffering mainly from reminiscences" (Freud 1893: 7) and indicates their potential relevance for solving the puzzling question as to why these shell shock patients are psychically fixated on their traumas (Freud 1920: 13; Fletcher 2013: 288ff).

This "reappearance" of hysteria in Freud's work is telling with regard to his continuous efforts at "conquering psychiatry."[68] In general, we can say that shifts and developments in Freud's psychoanalytic practice (case studies) and theory parallel major trends in German psychiatric literature. This fact has to be taken into account if we want to understand developments in Freud's writings after the publication of *Three Essays* in 1905. After 1905, Freud gets more and more followers and sympathizers, especially from the field of psychiatry – Carl Gustav Jung, Karl Abraham, Eugen Bleuler, Sandor Ferenczi, Abraham Brill, Ludwig Binswanger, and others (Binswanger 1920; Vandermeersch 1991; Falzeder 2007). Not only were they allies in Freud's wish to "conquer psychiatry," but they also developed theories of their own and brought to the fore their clinical material and expertise, to which Freud had to respond and which proved to be of great importance for the development of psychoanalysis.[69]

In a way, Freud had already paved the way for developments in the years after the publication of *Three Essays* in 1905. In a series of publications from the mid-1890s, Freud had proposed, based on his clinical experience and contrary to

Krafft-Ebing, that obsessional ideas and phobias were of psychic origin and should be detached from the category of neurasthenia. Given the fact that someone like Kraepelin had differentiated between neurasthenia and hysteria by arguing that in neurasthenia obsessional ideas take the place of contractions and paralyses (May-Tolzmann 1998: 341), one can see that Freud's proposal to detach obsessional ideas from neurasthenia moved in the vicinity of hysteria. In the mid-1890s, Freud had in fact become convinced that the "neuropsychoses of defence" consisted of four types (hysteria, obsessional neurosis, paranoia, and hallucinatory acute amentia or melancholia) that shared many characteristics, notably the fact that they were all pathological *psychic* states that could not be explained by reference to hereditary factors or physiological defects. In fact, it was the role played by sexuality (infantile sexual experience, excitation, pleasure/unpleasure, repression) in the etiology of these neuropsychoses of defense that defined these types as a family group (Freud 1894, 1895, 1898; May-Tolzmann 1998). From this, one can understand why it was unproblematic for Freud to engage in the study of the psychoses (dementia paranoides, dementia praecox, schizophrenia), phobias, obsessional neuroses, and later also melancholia,[70] in the years after the first publication of *Three Essays*.[71] For the later versions of that text, Freud's study of the psychoses – and his interactions notably with the Burghölzli group (Jung, Bleuler, Abraham, etc.) – is of particular importance.

In the years after 1905, Freud embarked on an intense correspondence and passionate debate with Jung about psychosis and the sexual nature of the libido. In 1907, Jung published his book on dementia praecox,[72] in which the memoirs of Senatspräsident Schreber are mentioned for the first time in the history of psychoanalytic thinking (Jung 1907; Vandermeersch 1991). Freud would return to these famous memoirs in his case study on Schreber, published in 1911, which contains his own most fully articulated theory of psychotic pathology (Freud 1911). The systematic reflection on psychosis that Freud began in his discussions with Jung confronted him with a problem for which the study of hysteria had not really prepared him. Indeed, psychosis confronted him with the fact that both the object and the ego supporting the relation to it can be absent, or can be lost in the course of our existence. Whereas hysteria taught Freud about the importance of sexuality for human existence, psychosis now informed him about the uncertain status of our relation to reality as such. Freud had no choice but to tackle this problem, but at the same time he did not want to give up the primacy of sexuality. At this point, the limitations of Freud's structural opposition between sexuality and food intake became obvious. Both Jung and Bleuler showed Freud that the "loss" of reality that characterizes psychosis refers to a dysfunction at the level of affectivity, or, in more contemporary terms, our affective attachment to the world and to others. This affective relation to reality obviously cannot be reduced to the narrow definition of self-preservation that Freud used in his texts. And since Freud acknowledged only two drives, he had no choice but to consider this relation essentially sexual. The conflicts with Jung over the libido theory, and with Alfred Adler over the nature of the ego in its function of relating to objects (through aggression, power), were born from this commitment. These discussions and considerations are crucial for understanding Freud's theoretical innovations, notably the introduction of narcissism and his formulation of a drive theory, which also found their way into the later editions of *Three Essays*. According to Freud himself, it was these innovations in particular that had created the possibility for a lasting contribution of psychoanalysis to the study and treatment of dementia praecox, paranoia, and melancholia, and as such they were thus crucial for the "conquering" of psychiatry (Freud 1919a).

While trying to "conquer psychiatry," Freud and his followers were also trying to apply psychoanalytic theory to cultural phenomena such as art, religion, and philosophy (Rank & Sachs 1912). Indeed, the decade between 1905 and 1915 is a period of explorations of new clinical and cultural territories, and some of the results of these explorations can be witnessed in the 1910 and 1915 editions of *Three Essays*. In the context of these explorations, it became clear that hysteria would not suffice to understand these cultural phenomena. In Freud's interpretation of religion (totemism) and morality (taboo), for instance, the father, aggression, guilt, and conscience formation all play key roles (Freud 1907, 1912–1913; Westerink 2009, 2017). However, these phenomena are not central themes in hysterical pathology. Since Freud remained faithful to his patho-analytic starting point, he had to turn to other psychopathologies to properly understand these crucial aspects of human life. Freud's shift of attention to obsessional neurosis is at least partly a result of this new interest; it is no coincidence that Freud's first text on obsessional neurosis was also a text on religious ceremonies (Freud 1907). Obsessional neurosis, Freud reasons, is indeed structured around the problem of aggression, guilt, and conscience.

With the introduction of obsessional neurosis as nosological category, Freud also expected to play a decisive role in the ongoing discussions in psychiatric literature regarding obsessional ideas as distinct from hallucinatory ideas (May-Tolzmann 1998). Psychiatry was a field with huge potential for a positive reception of psychoanalytic theory, methods, and practice, especially if psychoanalysis could contribute to the study of all the psychoneuroses. Hysteria alone did not allow Freud to turn psychoanalysis into the general theory he progressively wanted it to be.

Final remarks and outlook

The developments and innovations in the fields of neurology and psychiatry provided a strong motive for redirecting attention from hysteria to other psychopathologies and fields that promised to be important for the further advancement of psychoanalysis as theory and practice but also as a discipline with its own institutions (societies, journals) and its own secure place in an eminent medical field (psychiatry). But there were also intrinsic reasons why Freud had to reconsider his 1905 theory of sexuality and the paradigmatic status of hysteria. We already mentioned several inconsistencies and problems in the first edition of *Three Essays* that undermined Freud's overall picture of sexuality. He claims systematically in this first edition that infantile sexuality is autoerotic and without an object. He illustrates this claim by taking orality as a model. Oral symptoms indeed play a crucial role in hysterical symptomatology (hysterical vomiting, globus hystericus, etc.), which Freud had notably shown in the case study of Dora. But so does the voyeuristic drive for watching. Can we conceive this drive without referring to an object? At no point, however, do the limits of Freud's original model become clearer than they do with regard to the drive for mastery and the status of sadomasochism.[73] Like all other perversions, Freud tries to understand sadomasochism from the perspective of its leading erogenous zone and the partial drive to which it can be linked as well as the reaction formation that subsequently represses the pleasures that are caused by the satisfaction of the latter. Most importantly, it becomes obvious in Freud's treatment of this specific perversion that hysteria does not allow for a sufficient understanding of aggression. Indeed, aggression plays only a minor role in the symptomatology of hysteria. Freud himself refers to obsessional neurosis as a better candidate to articulate this problem (Freud 1905a: 29).

The main question the first edition of *Three Essays* left unanswered was how the transformation of puberty – the shift from a non-objectal infantile to an objectal adult sexuality – came about. In 1905, Freud tends to take the two organizations of sexuality – the infantile and the adult one – for granted. He implicitly seems to suggest that the transformations in puberty can be considered natural and normal in the way his predecessors had already articulated this: sexuality in the service of procreation only emerges "naturally" with the physical and psychical maturity of a person. With full development of the sexual organs and the production of sexual substances, creating sexual (adult) excitement, sexuality was first constituted. Freud's predecessors could therefore argue that the infant was a non-sexual being. But with the discovery of infantile sexuality, an explanation for the transition between the two regimes became an eminent issue. It is this issue that will determine the main changes seen in the later editions of *Three Essays*.

The next chapters are devoted to the introduction of various sections, passages, and footnotes in the later editions of *Three Essays* from 1910, 1915, 1920, and 1924. We will show that the various additions and alterations will indeed fundamentally undermine the original 1905 theory and its critique of the "poetic fable," i.e., the functional and heteronormative perspective on sexuality.

Notes

1 With regard to sexuality, Freud uses both the term *Geschlechtstrieb* and *Sexualtrieb*. *Geschlechtstrieb* can be translated as genital drive because it refers to the genitally organized sexual attraction between two individuals. *Sexualtrieb*, on the contrary, refers to Freud's new concept of sexuality that is no longer defined in terms of an intrinsic natural genital object. See also our later discussion.

2 Krafft-Ebing uses genital drive (*Geschlechtstrieb*), sexual drive (*Sexualtrieb*), and reproduction drive (*Fortpflanzungstrieb*) as equivalents; Freud does not.

3 On Krafft-Ebing and his influence on Freud, see Sulloway (1979), Oosterhuis (2000, 2012), and Davidson (2001).

4 Notably, in his 1871 *The Descent of Man*, Darwin had argued that nutrition and reproduction should be understood on the basis of the instinct for self-preservation. Darwin distinguishes this instinct from other fundamental instincts; namely, social instincts such

as "sympathy" and "love," especially as directed toward family members and beloved objects but also larger groups (communities, society) (Darwin 1981: 72ff;). Freud does not refer to a theory of sympathy in *Three Essays*. In later writings, he will explicitly reject the notion of a social instinct in favor of a theory of identification (Freud 1921: 117–121). On this issue, see also Westerink (2009: 124–126, 184–185).

5 Arnold Davidson has correctly argued that the distinction between normal (natural) and perverse (unnatural) sexuality was not a post-Darwinian invention of psychiatry and sexology. The distinction has much older roots in a long Western Christian tradition of a hermeneutics of sexual life continued into modern times. The shift that takes place in the nineteenth century consists of the reassignment of the study and regulation of the perversions from (a religiously motivated) morality and law to medicine – a shift that also includes a continuation of a strong moral evaluation of the perversions. It is only now that the perversions can be defined in terms of distinct pathologies and subjective identities (Davidson 2001: 23–24). On the same topic, see also Mazaleigue (2014).

6 This impulse mainly described what Freud calls "tender feelings" (*Zärtlichkeit*) and what we would today refer to as "attachment" (see later discussion). On the works of Moll, see Sauerteig (2012) and Sigusch (2012).

7 In his 1901 article, Krafft-Ebing further argues that in acquired homosexuality – the common form of homosexuality – seduction plays a decisive role. It is for this reason that suggestion can be a therapeutic tool in the cure of homosexuality. Given Freud's views on seduction (see later discussion) and the well-known response of Krafft-Ebing to Freud's lecture on the seduction theory in 1896, characterizing it as a scientific fairy tale, this reference to seduction is remarkable. However, we should also note that the German psychologist and sexologist Albert von Schrenck-Notzing had claimed that cultural factors such as education were decisive in the etiology of perversions, and that suggestion and hypnosis could be successfully employed in therapy (Oosterhuis 2000: 61, 2012).

8 We should note here that Freud mainly deals with homosexuality as a "perversion" and in doing so shows the fundamental shortcomings of the theoretical models of his predecessors. That does not mean that Freud's view of homosexuality as such is clear and consistent. In the 1905 edition, the paradigmatic form of homosexuality is the adult man's love of boys and young adolescents in ancient Greece. Some years later, in the Schreber case, Freud will argue that Schreber's transgender wish to become a woman can in fact be called a homosexual wish. But the identification of Greek pederasty or Schreber's transsexuality as homosexuality is far from self-evident (Freud 1905a: 9–10, 1911).

9 The implication is what Arnold Davidson has rightfully described as "a conceptually devastating blow to the entire structure of nineteenth-century theories of sexual psychopathology" (Davidson 2001: 79).

10 Freud tries to explain this development by drawing upon evolutionary developments: in starting to walk upright, man is estranged from the smells of the earth and former visual experiences. Shame and disgust are the first results of this evolutionary process, and as such they mark the first difference between man and animal. On organic repression, see Haute and Geyskens (2004: 44–45).

11 We are far removed here from the metapsychological theories on perversion that were developed after Freud and *in the name of* Freud. The reader may think here of the classical book by Stoller (1975) and of the work of Lacan. In both cases, "perversion" is thematized as a distinctive "identity" – calling it a structure (Lacan) does not change much in this context – that can be clearly distinguished from other identities ("structures"). In this respect, Freud is more on the side of recent queer theory than on the side of traditional psychoanalysis (Dean 2008; Haute 2016).

12 It seems that Freud calls pain a reaction formation because he is looking for an explanation of sadomasochism that is formally analogous to his explanation of the other perversions. Just as shame is a limit that is overcome in voyeurism/exhibitionism, so, too, is pain considered the limit that is overcome or put into question in sadomasochism. But

what forbidden pleasure could pain possibly hide? Freud's basic model of perversion is hard to universalize, and it cannot make the different perversions intelligible in the same way.

13 In his writings on hysteria, Freud occasionally thematizes a form of aggression that has no inherent object; namely, rage or anger. It is telling that in his studies of obsessional neurosis, Freud will highlight hatred (and the ambivalence of feelings) as being of fundamental importance for understanding all object-related forms of aggression, including sadism (Westerink 2016).

14 Freud would later recall that Charcot commented, with reference to the origin of hysteria, "C'est toujours la chose génitale, toujours . . . toujours . . . toujours" (Westerink 2009: 8).

15 In *Three Essays*, this development in Freud's thought is most clearly expressed in endnote 7: "[i]n the understanding of inversion, pathological approaches have been replaced by anthropological ones" (Freud 1905a: 91).

16 In German psychiatry, it was Otto Binswanger who in 1904 published a voluminous and influential handbook on hysteria (Binswanger 1904). In this book, he connects to the writings of predecessors such as Charcot and Moebius, while arguing that hysteria should be explained from a "psychopathic disposition," and that psychic dynamics merely influence the concrete manifestation of hysteria and are not to be regarded a factor in the etiology.

17 Rank and Sachs argued in their programmatic opening article in the first issue of *Imago* (1912) that because of Freud's view of the psychopathologies as magnifications and exaggerations of general human psychic dynamics, the findings derived from the study of psychopathologies could not be limited to the field of pathology alone. The step toward the study of normal everyday phenomena (dreams, jokes, slips of the tongue, and the like) and cultural phenomena such as art, myth, and religion could and should also be made. The latter phenomena were of particular interest in the field of applied psychoanalysis since, according to Rank and Sachs, these cultural phenomena could be regarded as theater staging those repressed drives that were apparently unusable (not functional) in practical cultural life. Hence, psychoanalysis was particularly interested in those cultural phenomena that did not contribute to the preservation of the individual and the group through procreation and labor (communal and family life). Two remarks should be made about this. First, this view of applied psychoanalysis as the study of "theatrical stages" is still closely associated with the model of hysteria and Freud's critique of the functional interpretation of the sexual drives. Second, the anthropological approach in *Three Essays* indeed enables this text to be situated in a series of attempts (starting with *Interpretation of Dreams*) to analyze general human aspects of everyday life (Rank & Sachs 1912).

18 In this context, Freud also remarks that "among the unconscious trains of thought found in neuroses, there is nothing corresponding to a tendency to fetishism." This shows us that the relation between the neuroses and the perversions is more complex than the formula "neurosis is the negative of perversion" at first sight seems to suggest (Freud 1905a: 26, 28).

19 This seems to parallel the kind of ambiguity and "need of variation" one also finds in bisexuality.

20 Freud adds in a footnote: "[i]t is scarcely possible to exaggerate the pathogenic significance of the comprehensive tie uniting the sexual and the excremental, a tie which is at the basis of a very large number of hysterical phobias" (Freud 1905d: 32).

21 Freud places "drive" in quotation marks, and with good reason: in 1905 he had not yet formulated a drive theory. To support an interpretation of the drive as (the/a?) motor impulse, one might refer to *Project of a Scientific Psychology* (1895), where Freud had developed a neurobiological theory of stimuli (*Reize*) and pressure (*Drang*) in terms of the quantities and discharges of neurons (Freud 1950). However, the *Project* was never published during Freud's lifetime, and we find no references to this theory in *Three Essays*.

22 Why did Freud delete this passage in 1915? An important reason can be found in Jung's exposition of his genetic theory of the libido (1912a), which offers yet another peculiar reading of the passage. Jung argues that Freud suggests a single primordial drive splitting up in various directions and causing certain bodily functions, zones, and objects to be cathected with sexuality. In this way, zones (for example, the lips) that were initially without sexual function could receive such a function (kissing) in the context of a natural process of efficient differentiation and growth. In this reading, the drive does not become sexual through the link with bodily zones; on the contrary, certain bodily zones receive a sexual function when the primordial libido differentiates into various domains and specialized functions. It is against Jung's genetic theory of the drives that Freud will then stress the existence of two primal drives, one of which is sexual by nature and aimed at preservation of the species. To prevent any misunderstanding and future heresies, he deletes the passage. See Jung (1912a: 133–139) and Vandermeersch (1991: 231ff, 2017).

23 Because of his critique of the functional approach in contemporary Darwinian thought, Freud basically dismisses all arguments for the Darwinian drive dichotomy. Interestingly, Freud does not provide any new arguments for the idea that psychic life is characterized by two fundamental tendencies or drives.

24 There could be another argument that Freud does not develop in the text we are commenting on: the infantile pleasures are clearly sexual when they are integrated into adult sexuality (e.g., kissing). Since they are "sexual" at the end of the development, they must already have been sexual from the beginning.

25 This probably also explains why Freud, in discussing the "sources of infantile sexuality" at the end of the second part of his text, identifies without much ado the pleasurable experiences caused by "mechanical vibrations" (one could think here of sitting in a train) as sexual in nature. Along the same lines, Freud writes that intellectual activities can go along with "a concomitant sexual excitation," which "is no doubt the only justifiable basis for what is in other respects a highly questionable derivation of nervous disturbances from intellectual 'overwork'" (Freud 1905a: 54, 57).

26 We do not agree with Jonathan Lear's reading of Freud's theory on infantile sexuality (Lear 2005: 70–82). Lear argues that in Freud's view, human sexuality is essentially imaginative and that sensual sucking is a pleasurable imaginative activity. We find a similar idea in the work of Jean Laplanche (1987: 71). According to Laplanche, the infantile autoerotic activity is essentially phantasmatic. According to Freud, however, neither imagination nor phantasy is among pleasurable infantile activities.

27 Ulrike May-Tolzmann has shown that it is only in the 1915 edition of *Three Essays* that Freud will first associate sensual sucking with the aim of "incorporation of the object" (cannibalistic tendencies, introjection, identification). Hence, it is in 1915 that Freud reinterprets sensual sucking in object-relational terms (May-Tolzmann 2015a: 134–142).

28 "In childhood, therefore, the sexual drive is without an object, that is, *autoerotic*" (Freud 1905a: 82).

29 One could think here, for instance, of Lacan's famous dictum that "desire is lack of being" (Lacan 1966: 793–827).

30 "A young man who was a great admirer of feminine beauty was talking once – so the story went – of the good-looking wet-nurse who had suckled him when he was a baby: 'I'm sorry,' he remarked, 'that I did not make a better use of my opportunity.' I was in the habit of quoting this anecdote to explain the factor of deferred action in the mechanism of the psychoneurosis" (Freud 1900: 204–205).

31 In later texts – and especially in the study on the Wolf Man – Freud no longer links deferred action (*Nachträglichkeit*) to puberty. On this issue, see Laplanche 2006.

32 On the notion of *Nachträglichkeit* in the work of Freud, see Laplanche 2006 and Fletcher 2013.

33 Albert Moll argues that the concept of *Trieb* should not be used to describe all contingent psychic movements, intentions, strivings, and acts of the will – as, for example, Wilhelm Wundt had argued – but instead should be used to denote the psychic

disposition that pushes a person to perform a certain act. This raises the question of the distinction between *Trieb* and *Instinkt*. Moll argues that the *Geschlechtstrieb* – the instinct aimed at coitus and intimacy with an adult partner of the opposite sex – is merely the conscious and subjective side of an unconscious *Fortpflanzunsinstinkt* that has reproduction as its goal. Although *Trieb* and *Instinkt* are thus two dimensions of the same process, Moll prefers to use the concept of *Trieb* precisely because of its subjective side, i.e., its relevance for an understanding of the psychological aspects of sexuality, such as sexual satisfaction, attachment, and object choice (Moll 1898: 1–8).

34 For this reason, Strachey's decision to translate *Trieb* as "instinct" can be defended against the critique based on a distinction between nature (animal, biological processes) and culture (human, psychological dynamics) we find, for example, in Lacanian theory.

35 In Strachey's translation of *Three Essays*, this distinction is completely blurred by the fact that Strachey translates both concepts as "sexual instinct."

36 One can think here, for instance, of Ernst Kris, who writes the following: "[i]n his letters [to Wilhelm Fliess], we learn that Freud's insight into the structure of the Oedipus complex, that is, the core problem of psychoanalysis, was made possible by his self-analysis, which he began in the summer of 1897 during his stay in Aussee" (Kris 1952: 545, our translation). This argumentation has become "classic" and has continued in key publications until the present day. See, for example, Gay (1988) and Phillips (2014). The latter writes the following: "[b]ecause sexuality begins as incestuous desire for the parents – as Freud was discovering what he took to be his own and everyone else's Oedipus complex in his self-analysis – it terrorizes us" (Ibid.: 107).

37 We will return to this problem in more detail in our third chapter.

38 We have to read this statement together with another one from "My Views" that seems to contradict it: "[a]t that time my material was still scanty, and it happened by chance to include a proportionately large number of cases in which sexual seduction by an adult or by older children played the chief part in the history of the patient's childhood. I thus overestimated the frequency of such events (though in other respects they were not open to doubt)" (Freud 1906: 152). The contradiction is only apparent. What Freud says is that he did not overestimate the importance of seduction in the eighteen cases he reported in "The Aetiology of Hysteria." But since he did not realize at that time that sexual constitution can also arouse a child's sex life, he overestimated its importance in general. For this interpretation and for a more detailed reading of these passages, see Davidson (1984).

39 For a more detailed account, see Haute 2018.

40 The few references to this complex were introduced in later editions and more particularly in the footnotes to the edition of 1920. See chapter 3.

41 It is only in the edition of 1915 that Freud describes infantile sexuality as objectal in itself. From that time forward, he speaks of a "diphasic object choice." The first phase would take place in the period between two and five years old. The object choices of that period would appear "unutilizable" because of repression and then be inhibited until their return at the beginning of puberty (Freud 1905c: 200).

42 It seems clear from the context that the "interests" we need to build a community are, according to Freud, of a libidinal nature, but Freud does not explain – or is not yet capable of explaining – in the first edition of *Three Essays* how the transformation of the libidinal investment of the parental figures gives rise to social feelings. The establishment of social bonds is not thematized in this text. It is not until *Totem and Taboo* (1912–1913) that Freud will provide a full account of this thematic.

43 "His fate moves us only because it might have been our own, because the oracle laid upon us before our birth the very curse which rested upon him" (Freud 1900: 246–247).

44 Freud further systematized the insights he gained from these studies in some new paragraphs on "the sexual researches of children" that he will add to the 1915 edition of his text. He concludes from the case of Little Hans that the process of the choice of object is "diphasic" and occurs in two waves, the first taking part in the period between two and five years, the second setting in with puberty (1905c: 200). Pubertal and adult

sexuality can only now be considered the "persistence" and "revival" of the infantile object choices. The 1915 paragraph on the diphasic object choice thus marks a fundamental shift in Freud's thinking on sexuality. No longer does he defend a strict dichotomy between an autoerotic infantile period and an object-related adult sexuality (Freud 1905c: 194–200).

45 The idea that the Oedipus complex contains the key to *all* psychopathology – meaning that all psychopathological syndromes are to be considered vicissitudes of the (psychosexual) relations between the child and its parents, and that this is the obligatory road for entry into the world of culture – is first formulated in the fourth essay of *Totem and Taboo* (Freud 1912–1913: 160–161). The Oedipus complex gets its canonical formulation in *The Ego and the Id* of 1923, in which Freud calls it the shibboleth of psychoanalysis (Freud 1923b: 13).

46 We find similar attachment behavior in other primates even if they do not have as long a period of dependency on the mother as humans do (Bowlby 1969).

47 "We can anticipate that these characteristics will be found to apply to most of the other activities of the infantile sexual drive" (Freud 1905a: 43).

48 This explains why, in the beginning of the third part, Freud qualifies infantile sexuality as "*predominantly* autoerotic" (Ibid.: 61, emphasis ours).

49 A reason for this imbalance could be the fact that in *Three Essays* Freud takes hysteria as the model for the study of sexuality. In earlier writings, he had associated cruelty almost exclusively with the obsessional neurotic's aggressive urge for sexual pleasure. Another reason lies in the fact that Freud clearly wants to relate his text to Krafft-Ebing's catalog of the various sexual perversions.

50 In this quotation, Freud seems to identify "love" and "sexual need" (*Sexualbedürfnis*), an identification that is far from self-evident. But the status of "love" is difficult to thematize within the exclusive distinction between sexuality and self-preservation.

51 This does not mean, however, that Freud gives a determinative role to the sexuality of the adult in the constitution of infantile sexuality, as Laplanche does. The child responds to the adult's initiative, but this response originates exclusively in the child. Freud remains an "ipsocentrist."

52 In this context, we can also begin to understand Freud's reference to Little Hans as "a little Oedipus": Hans responds to the loving care of his mother with a wish for intimate contact by sleeping beside her and thus gaining pleasure from skin contact. For this reason, he develops a wish to have his father "out of the way." In this train of thought, the hostility toward the father develops from a sexual aim that is still essentially autoerotic (pleasure derived from cutaneous contact) (Freud 1909a: 111).

53 "The normality of sex life is warranted solely by an exact convergence of the two currents directed toward the sexual object and the sexual aim. . . . The sexual drive now puts itself at the service of the reproductive function" (Freud 1905a: 61).

54 In the summary of the text, Freud writes that puberty brings about the primacy of the genital zone and the finding of the object. The latter is immediately identified with a heterosexual object (Freud 1905a: 83). Interestingly enough, Freud adds that the object choice is prepared in the infantile period by the "sexual inclination" of children toward their parents and caregivers, which is refreshed at the beginning of puberty, and by the introduction of the incest barriers that turn children away from these objects. Does this not also undermine the general line of Freud's argumentation by introducing a more "functional approach" to sexuality? And does this not anticipate, albeit in an extremely sketchy way, later developments, such as the Oedipus complex?

55 Freud conceives of sexuality in this first edition to a large extent without any reference to sexual difference. The problematic of sexual difference only comes to the fore at the beginning of puberty, when sexuality finds its object. The introduction of this difference is, moreover, immediately linked to the different roles the sexes play in reproduction: "[s]ince the new sexual aim assigns very different functions to the two sexes, their sexual development now diverges widely" (Freud 1905a: 61). Clearly, Freud here surrenders to the paradigm of classical sexology.

56 "I have recently been able to throw light upon another example, from a vastly different area of psychical dynamics, in which similarly, a greater effect of pleasure is being afforded by means of a less intense sensation of pleasure acting, as it were, as an incentive bonus. This also provided an opportunity to take a closer look at the nature of pleasure" (Freud 1905a: 65).
57 "That being so, it cannot be disputed that we supplement our pleasure by attaining the laughter that is impossible for us by the roundabout path of the impression we have of the person who has been made to laugh. As Dugas has put it, we laugh as it were 'par ricochet.' . . . When I make the other person laugh by telling him my joke, I am actually making use of him to arouse my own laughter" (Freud 1905b: 155–156).
58 For an extensive and brilliant interpretation of the passages we are commenting on here, see Moyaert (2012).
59 At this point, our reading of the 1905 *Three Essays* as a text in which Freud identifies two regimes of sexuality – infantile autoerotic sexuality and pubertal/adult genital object-related sexuality – comes close to Laplanche's reading of *Three Essays* (Laplanche 2007). We would like to note, however, that although Laplanche acknowledges the significance of the distinction made by Freud between *Sexualtrieb* (sexual drive) and *Geschlechtstrieb* (genital drive), he doesn't interpret the *Sexualtrieb* in the same way as we do here. Laplanche opposes the *pulsion sexuelle* (*Sexualtrieb*) to the *pulsion sexué* (*Geslechtstrieb*). What he calls "sexual" refers to the sexual unconscious that consists of that part of the enigmatic (sexual) messages of the other that couldn't be translated (integrated) by the little child. Hence, the Laplanchean "sexual" does not correspond to the autoerotic in the Freudian sense (Laplanche 2007: 153–175).
60 This reference to the theater and, hence, culture inevitably introduces the psychoanalytic problem of sublimation that Freud also mentions in his text without paying much attention to it. In this text, Freud considers sublimation within the context, or even as a subcategory, of the reaction formation (Freud 1905a: 38–39).
61 "But the limits of such disgust are purely conventional; a man who passionately kisses the lips of a pretty girl may be disgusted at the idea of using her toothbrush, even though there are no grounds for supposing that his own oral cavity, for which he feels no disgust, is any cleaner than that of the girl" (Freud 1905a: 14).
62 In Freud's view, culture cannot but take nature into account and respect its fundamental tendencies: "[e]ducation will remain perfectly within its mandated domain if it limits itself to following the lines which have already been laid down organically, and to imprinting them somewhat more clearly and deeply" (Freud 1905a: 39).
63 As early as 1890, Freud writes the following: "[i]t is not until we have studied pathological phenomena that we can get an insight into normal ones" (Freud 1890: 286).
64 On Freud's conflicting views on sexuality in the 1905 *Three Essays*, see also Blass (2017).
65 This is notably the case with neurasthenia – a concept that in the 1890s Krafft-Ebing had described as a pathological change in the central nervous system due to increased stress and pressure on a person in modern society (Westerink 2009: 64–67).
66 The concept of traumatic neurosis was introduced in German literature in 1889 by the neurologist Hermann Oppenheim, who had used the diagnosis for injured (brain damage) industrial workers. This conception of traumatic neurosis was rejected in favor of a psychogenic approach to the shell shock phenomenon at a conference held in 1916 by German neurologists and psychiatrists in Munich. Instead, the concept of war neurosis became more generally used to refer to a disorder in which older concepts merged, notably traumatic neurosis, psychoneurosis (as defined in psychoanalysis), hysteria, and concepts of constitutional inferiority. These concepts continued to be used until after World War II (Kloocke, Schmiedebach & Priebe 2005).
67 Kraepelin had prepared the ground for this interpreation when he categorized hysteria, together with neurasthenia and traumatic neurosis, as a psychogenic pathology (Kraepelin 1915; Weber 2015).
68 In 1906 Freud writes the following to Bleuler: "I am confident that we will soon conquer psychiatry" (Schröter 2012: 100).

69 Freud discusses and describes this evolution himself in "On the History of the Psycho-analytic Movement" (Freud 1914b).
70 The opening passage of Freud's 1917 text on melancholia shows that his aim is to make a contribution to psychiatry. Contrary to Kraepelin (1915), who had listed melancholia under the category of endogenic pathologies, Freud proposes to view melancholia – like hysteria and obsessional neurosis – as a psychogenic pathology (Freud 1917).
71 In late nineteenth-century psychiatric literature, the concept of psychosis was mostly used as a general term indicating mental illness (*Geisteskrankheiten*) and sometimes also as a synonym for the psychoneuroses (or neuropsychoses) (Beer 1995). It was only in the later editions of Kraepelin's and Jasper's textbooks – and, hence, after Freud's Schreber case – that a systematic distinction between the neuroses and psychoses was made.
72 In *Über die Psychologie der Dementia Praecox*, Jung strongly focuses on the similarities between hysteria and dementia praecox, thus assuming a connection between the two, which was also promising for further psychoanalytic inquiry. In the same period, Karl Abraham published several articles on the same topic, notably "Die psychosexuellen Differenzen der Hysterie und der Dementia Praecox" (1908). On this issue, see also May-Tolzmann (2015a: 101–125).
73 One should also mention fetishism in this context (Freud 1905a: 16–17). We return to this issue in the next chapter.

2

THE INFANT'S OBJECT CHOICE AND DEVELOPMENT

Introduction

In the previous chapter, we identified several extrinsic and intrinsic reasons why Freud inserted so much new theoretical material in the text that did not support or complement the original theory. We already mentioned that the main question the first edition of *Three Essays* left unanswered was how the transformation of puberty – the shift from a non-objectal infantile to an objectal adult sexuality – came about. Notably, this problem incited Freud to progressively introduce in the later editions of *Three Essays* a developmental approach that was almost completely absent from the first edition. This approach is introduced through two perspectives that are clearly linked and yet also distinct. In the years after 1905, Freud looks for empirical evidence that would support his theories on infantile sexuality. He expects to find this evidence in his case analysis of Little Hans and in the analyses of infantile sexual researches and theories related to this case (1908a, 1909a) (for example, the case of a non-hysterical but phobic patient) and in exploring a drive – the drive for knowledge (*Wißtrieb*) – that had not been mentioned in the 1905 *Three Essays*. In these studies of as yet unexplored terrain, Freud realizes that the relation between infantile sexuality and the finding of an object is much more complex than he initially thought. In line with these new findings, Freud develops the idea of a diphasic introduction of the object of sexuality, which replaces the original distinction between a non-objectal and objectal regime. It is no coincidence that, for the first time, Freud mentions the Oedipus complex *qua complex* in 1910 (Freud 1910a: 47), and indeed one could argue that it was the studies of Little Hans and infantile sexual theories that prepared ground for the introduction of this complex. After all, the Oedipus complex presupposes the idea that the infant has an interest in objects (persons) and their sexual life.[1] In the 1915 version of *Three Essays*, the introduction of the idea of the diphasic object choice equally prepares the references to the Oedipus complex that are introduced – albeit only in footnotes – in the fourth edition published in 1920 onward.[2] In the next chapter, we will explore the question as to why Freud could not or did not want to introduce the Oedipus complex in a more substantial form than merely footnotes.

Meanwhile, the study of psychosis, and more particularly of Schreber's *Weltuntergangserlebnis* ("the imminence of a great catastrophe, of the end of the world") (Freud 1911: 68), confronted Freud with the fact that the relation of the ego and the object cannot be taken for granted. In other words, psychosis showed Freud that the relation between the ego and the object is not automatically installed. In this context, he first introduces the concept of narcissism, indicating a developmental phase between autoerotism and object choice. This developmental approach and the related issue of narcissism are explicitly thematized in new paragraphs on "developmental phases and the sexual organization" and "the libido theory" in which Freud first places the different erogenous zones on a timeline so that each of them gets a specific role in the constitution of the (relation to the) object.

In the present chapter, we will first discuss in detail the problems Freud had already encountered in his discussion of sadomasochism in 1905. We will also mention the problems he comes across with regard to fetishism since they are of a similar kind as those related to sadomasochism. The analysis of these perversions appearing in the subsequent editions of *Three Essays* will allow us to convincingly show the limits of Freud's paradigmatic model of hysteria. We will then present the introduction of the developmental approach in Freud's thinking along the lines that we just mentioned. In doing so, we will show how these additions to the 1910 and 1915 editions fundamentally change the theory of sexuality developed in the 1905 *Three Essays*. The footnotes from 1920 on the Oedipus complex are completely in line with this tendency. The final result of this turn from a developmental perspective on the "normal" route toward adult object choice is this: from a trenchant critique of the contemporary sexology, *Three Essays* eventually turns into the justification of the "popular opinion"; that is, of the "instinctual" and functional interpretation of sexuality. We end this chapter with an analysis of the references to phylogenesis, biology, and homosexuality that Freud adds in the later edition and that are intrinsically linked to his new developmental approach.

The problem of sadomasochism

Three Essays contains several passages in which Freud discusses the status of sadomasochism. We know that Freud inherits the categorization of the different perversions from Krafft-Ebing. Freud not only repeats Krafft-Ebing's categories but also follows his descriptions of sadomasochism. For Krafft-Ebing, sadomasochism is not so much about pain, but submission. He further argues that sadism and masochism are two sides of the same coin: a masochist is always also a sadist and vice versa (Krafft-Ebing 1886: 140–143). At least in the first edition of *Three Essays*, Freud agrees with Krafft-Ebing on these two crucial issues. He stresses that pain is not what the sadomasochist is aiming at.[3] Quite the contrary, as we underscored in the previous chapter, he compares pain with the reaction formations of shame and disgust. This is already a first indication that Freud wants to understand sadomasochism within the framework of his hysterical paradigm. The development of shame and disgust is indeed at the basis of the repression of perverted tendencies – the oral drive and the drive for watching – that condition hysterical symptomatology. Just as shame and disgust limit the realization of these tendencies, so, too, does pain supposedly limit the tendency to submit oneself to the other or to the pleasurable submission of the other. But this analogy immediately appears highly problematic. The shame that we experience and that inhibits us from showing ourselves naked, for example, hides its opposite; namely, the pleasurable tendency to show ourselves naked in front of the other. This is why Freud calls neurosis the negative of perversion. But what exactly could be hiding "behind" the pain we feel or that we inflict on the other? Is not pain just what it is – pain? Pain has a limiting function but not in the same way shame and disgust have. Pain is an unpleasurable sensation that does not originate from a pleasurable sensation. Further in the text, Freud also mentions compassion as a possible *analogon* to shame and disgust (Freud 1905a: 52). This clearly makes more sense because an exaggerated compassion can hide an exaggerated tendency to physically or psychically harm the other.

But Freud develops the analogy much further than this. With regard to masochism, he refers in the 1905 edition to the psychological overvaluation of the object, which is itself linked to the anatomical extensions that we discussed in the previous chapter and that are a central aspect of Freud's explanation of hysteria. Humans ascribe all kinds of perfections to their love objects, and they diminish themselves in front of them: "you are everything to me; I am nothing compared to you." In the first edition, Freud considers masochism as nothing but an exaggeration of this tendency and thus as an exaggeration of an essentially hysterical mechanism – that is, the overvaluation of the love object in puberty and adult life (Ibid.: 20).[4] These passages disappear from the 1915 edition. They are replaced by a paragraph in which masochism is interpreted as sadism turned against oneself, which implies that masochism can now also be situated in infantile life. Completely in line with the positions he defends in "Instincts and Their Vicissitudes," also published in 1915, Freud thinks that masochism is always secondary and that it builds on a more originary sadism. In this context, Freud no longer refers to psychological overvaluation to explain masochism, but instead now writes that clinical analysis of extreme cases of masochism reveals the combined influence of a great number of factors that exaggerate and fixate the originally passive sexual attitude (castration complex, guilt). Even if Freud does not explain how exactly we should understand this remark, it is clear that masochism is no longer associated with a hysterical mechanism, and hence this new perspective relativizes the importance of the original hysterical model.

In both the 1905 and 1915 editions, sadism is interpreted as a magnified form of the aggressive component of the libido. In other words, Freud inserts these passages into his patho-analytic approach: sadism shows us in an exaggerated form something that is characteristic of human sexuality as such – its sadistic component.

According to Freud, this component of the libido is linked to the drive for mastery. In 1905, Freud maintained that this drive for mastery is not immediately sexual. As such, he did not have to reconsider the idea that infantile sexuality is essentially autoerotic. The drive for mastery gets sexualized through a process of "anastomosis," Freud writes in 1905. It is not immediately clear how this process should be understood. In the paragraph on the sources of infantile sexuality, Freud gives a hint to solve this problem. He mentions muscular activity ("bonding") as a possible source of the sadistic drive. Many people report that they first felt genital excitation while playfully fighting with others. Freud concludes: "[w]e might recognize one of the roots of the sadistic drive in the enhancement of sexual excitation by muscular activity" (Ibid.: 55). Freud does not change the passages on muscular activity in 1915, but in this third edition he no longer refers to anastomosis to explain the sexualization of the drive for mastery. Quite the contrary, he now considers this drive to be an intrinsic element of sexuality. The drive for mastery is essentially integrated into a sadistic component of the sexual drive. In the 1915 edition, Freud regards the sadistic impulses as both sexual from the beginning and as structurally directed toward an object. This implies that in the third edition Freud gave up his attempts to keep his analysis of sadomasochism in line with his original theory of infantile sexuality and, more particularly, that he puts in perspective the "hysterical" model of orality – the "lips kissing themselves" – to understand and qualify it.

In the first edition of his text, Freud stated that one of the most peculiar characteristics of sadomasochism is the fact that its active and passive forms *regularly* occur in one and the same person (Ibid.: 20).[5] In 1915, Freud replaces the adverb *regularly* with *always* (Freud 1905c: 159). He probably introduced this change simply to make the paragraph in which it occurs more consistent. Indeed, a few lines later in the 1905 version, he had already stated that a sadist is *always* to a greater or lesser degree a masochist and the other way around (Freud 1905a: 20). Freud here is a true student of Krafft-Ebing. He also follows Krafft-Ebing (1886: 140–143) – and not just Wilhelm Fliess, as he suggests himself – in linking this phenomenon in all the different editions of the text to bisexuality, in which masculinity (activity) and femininity (passivity) are said to be reconciled (Freud 1905c: 160). Just as in the case of psychic overvaluation, Freud here uses the conceptuality he had developed to understand hysteria for his explanation of sadomasochism.

However, this reference to bisexuality does not solve all the problems Freud is facing here. He writes in this context: "[a] person who feels pleasure in causing pain to someone else in a sexual relation is also capable of enjoying as pleasure any pain which he may himself derive from sexual relations" (Freud 1905a: 20). The reference to bisexuality is obviously not sufficient to understand this phenomenon. At the very least, we would need a theory of identification and of phantasy to explain the possibility of this reversal. But *Three Essays* contains no such a theory.[6] In this regard, Freud is correct to say about sadomasochism "that no satisfactory explanation of this perversion has been provided" (Ibid.).

Let us further develop our analysis of sadomasochism in *Three Essays*. Freud links the partial drives that are at the basis of the perversions to specific erogenous zones. The situation will be similar with regard to sadomasochism. As he notes in 1905, we have known since Jean-Jacques Rousseau that the passive drive for cruelty has its erogenous sources in the painful excitation of the skin of the buttocks. In the paragraph on the sources of infantile sexuality, he also formulates the hypothesis that the erogenous effect of painful sensations is at the origin of the sadomasochistic drive. Finally, Freud writes:

> [n]evertheless, in the sexual pleasure derived from watching, and in exhibitionism, the eye corresponds to an erogenous zone; while in the case of the components of the sexual drive which involves pain and cruelty, the same role is assumed by the skin, which in particular parts of the body has become differentiated into sense organs and modified into mucous membrane, and is thus the erogenous zone par excellence.
>
> *(Ibid.: 29–30)*

The reference to the skin as the erogenous zone of sadomasochism is thus much more ambiguous and less certain than in other cases. Freud seems to hesitate between the skin and the painful sensations of the skin. As Freud himself acknowledges in a footnote from 1924, the latter hypothesis seems to hint at the possibility of a primary *erogenous* masochism that cannot be reduced to a secondary masochism (sadism turned against oneself), which was given no attention in the earlier editions (Freud 1905c: 204, in note).

The discussion of sadomasochism in *Three Essays* remains in many respects uncertain, and this uncertainty is linked to the limits of the hysterical model Freud leaves behind beginning with the 1915 edition. Freud himself articulates the limits of this model with regard to sadomasochism. He claims that the role of the erogenous zones is quite clear in hysteria but much less so in other psychopathologies, such as obsessional neurosis and paranoia. In these pathologies, the formation of symptoms takes place in regions of the psychic apparatus that are much more removed from the body. Freud further states that obsessional neurosis might be much more suitable for the analysis of impulses that create new sexual goals and that are independent of erogenous zones (Freud 1905a: 29). Given the importance for the understanding of the obsessional neurosis of aggression and of the anal-sadistic pre-genital organization that Freud introduced in the 1915 edition, one is probably justified in thinking that hysteria is not the most suitable model to study sadomasochism.[7]

The problem of fetishism

Fetishism, Freud writes, is a very common characteristic of human sexuality. The "psychologically necessary overvaluation of the sexual object" can and will be transferred to anything that is related to this object (Ibid.: 17). Fetishism is thus an integral part of human sexuality, and explaining it is an urgent task for every theory of sexuality. But just as sadomasochism did, so, too, does fetishism put Freud's hysterical model and his ideas on infantile sexuality to the test.

Fetishism does not seem to fit in Freud's categorization of the sexual aberrations. It cannot be unambiguously considered either an aberration with regard to the sexual object or an aberration with regard to the sexual aim. Since its object is disconnected from reproduction, one would think that it is similar to homosexuality and pedophilia and hence an aberration with regard to the object. At the same time, fetishism implies the substitution of an overvalued sexual object for some part of the object's body or an inanimate object associated with that object that is inappropriate for normal sexual actions (union of the genitals). In this way, fetishism is also an aberration with regard to the "normal" sexual aim and is completely out of scope in the most extreme cases (Ibid.: 16).

In the 1905 edition, Freud explicitly refers to Alfred Binet, who first coined the term for his explanation of this phenomenon (Binet 1887).[8] According to Binet, fetishism had to be understood from the perspective of an accidental concurrence and subsequently enduring association between a powerful optical impression of a part of another person's body (hair, eyes, nails, feet, clothing, etc.) and sexual excitement. Freud seems to affirm this position: "[a]s Binet first claimed [. . .] the choice of fetish reveals the continuing influence of a sexual impression *mostly received in early childhood*, comparable with the proverbial 'stickiness' of first love under normal circumstances" (Freud 1905a: 17, emphasis ours). But how can we reconcile this idea with Freud's claim that infantile sexuality is essentially autoerotic? Does not the reference to Binet's views on fetishism imply that Freud would have to assume that the sexual drive is oriented toward the world of objects and their "impressions" from the start?

But this is not all. Freud claims that the different perversions manifest different partial drives in an exaggerated form. These partial drives are themselves linked to different erogenous zones and can best be studied in the infantile period (Ibid.: 32–33). But if they supposedly manifest themselves in fetishism, what could these partial drives be? Freud refers in this context to our tendency to "overvalue" our sexual objects. However, overvaluation of the object is not a partial drive, but rather a process that characterizes adult sexuality. And if infantile sexuality is essentially autoerotic, then it clearly makes no sense to speak of an erogenous zone that would be linked to the overvaluation of the object. It seems that both sadomasochism – "the most common and the most significant of all the perversions" (Ibid.: 19) – and fetishism cannot be explained in terms of the model that Freud defends in the first edition of *Three Essays*. Or, in other words, Freud is unable to relate fetishism to infantile sexuality, just as he was unable to relate masochism to infantile sexuality in 1905; consequently, he can provide an explanation only within the logic of adult sexuality (the overvaluation of a sexual object).

Infantile sexual researches and theories

In the preface to the 1910 edition of *Three Essays*, Freud states that he has resisted the temptation to introduce important psychoanalytic research results from the intervening five years in the text and instead prefers to preserve the "unity" of the

1905 theory of sexuality despite some unresolved issues and open questions. He mentions limiting himself to adding a few footnotes (Freud 1905c: 130). A footnote added to the paragraph about the partial drives in the second essay is particularly worth considering (Ibid.: 193–194). Here Freud writes that the 1905 theory of infantile sexuality was actually grounded in psychoanalytic research of adults – hysterical patients such as Dora – and hence this theory was not yet substantiated by empirical evidence to be found in the analysis of children. In the preceding years, the analysis of some cases of neurotic illness during the early years of childhood – notably the case study of Little Hans's phobia – had offered some empirical confirmation of his theoretical insights. However, Freud adds that his study of Little Hans had also produced some other, rather unexpected insights. The case study had actually shown "that children between the ages of three and five are capable of every clear object choice, accompanied by strong affects" (Ibid.: 194). Little Hans thus confronted Freud with a fundamental problem in his theory of sexuality concerning the conceptual and temporal separation of the phases of autoerotism and object love, or, in other words, the theory of sexuality that distinguished two clearly distinct sexual regimes – infantile and adult.

The case of Little Hans not only helped Freud identify and articulate this fundamental "defect" but also provided other valuable insights that helped him develop a first perspective on the transition from autoerotic to objectal sexuality. These insights concern first of all the importance of sexual research, investigations, inquiries, and theories of children and the consequent impact of these on developments in the sexual life of children.

In the 1915 edition, the 1910 footnote is replaced by a section on children's sexual research that, together with the newly added section on the developmental phases of sexual organization, provides two different perspectives on developments in early childhood. The focus in the section on children's sexual research is not so much on the direct exploration of the child's earliest object choices and object love as such, but rather on the question of what factors contribute to establishing the primacy of the genitals with regard to both its significance for the organization of infantile sexuality and its role in identifying objects as persons with genitals of their own. According to Freud, both factors can be considered preconditions for further development (the knowledge of sexual difference and the "normal" organization of adult sexuality in the service of reproduction).

Regarding children's sexual research – the questions they ask, their desire to see others' genitals, their tentative experiments – Freud writes in 1915 that "at about the same time as the sexual life of children reaches its first peak, between the ages of three and five, they begin to show signs of the activity which may be ascribed to the instinct [drive] for knowledge or research" (Ibid.: 194). He argues that this drive for knowledge only partly belongs to the sphere of sexuality. It makes use of the energy of the pleasure derived from watching (*Schaulust*), i.e., the sexual excitation through visual impressions, notably of the sexual object's hidden parts (Ibid.: 156). Yet the drive for knowledge itself does not originate from the sexual drive. It is "aroused under the goad of the self-seeking instincts [drives] that dominate him" (Freud 1908a: 212). This drive for knowledge is triggered by the first really big problem of life – the disturbing intrusion of a newborn sibling and the fear of loss of the parents' care and its potentially life-threatening implications. The desire for knowledge is thus not aimed at insight into random causal relations between things in the outside world but at finding a solution to a very acute and disturbing problem that takes the form of the question "Where do babies come from?" (Ibid.: 213).

According to Freud, the child clearly has some clue as to where babies come from since it notices the physical changes during the pregnancy of its mother. However, the child is and remains fundamentally ignorant about the existence of the vagina and the fertilizing role of semen (Ibid.: 214, 1905c: 196–197). The child is also ignorant about the meaning of coitus. When witnessing the sexual intercourse of the parents, the child interprets it as an act of ill-treatment or subjugation. This ignorance and misunderstanding are due to the fact that the interest in others does not emerge from the observation of sexual difference; nor does sexual difference constitute an acutely distressing problem for the child.[9] It is because the child is ignorant in this matter that his search for an answer to the one riddle that disturbs him – "Where do babies come from?" – will in the end be in vain. That is, the child will construct inadequate theories that link conception and birth to activities it does know; namely, eating and defecating. Hence, the first theories about adult sexuality are misinterpretations resulting from the infantile sexual constitution and the child's own polymorphous perverse activities. In infantile sexual theories, this is reflected in ideas about babies being born from the breast or navel or through the anus "like a discharge of faeces."

From this we can understand why Freud refers to this childhood research as "sexual" research. The question "Where do babies come from?" is not sexual in itself. The question has no relation to an autoerotic zone or pleasure; it merely reflects an "egoistic interest." But according to Freud, the child in search of an answer to this "egoistic" question is guided by the autoerotic components that inform the search for knowledge. The child's answers to the question of where babies come from draw upon the polymorphous perverse autoerotism that defines infantile sexual life. It is for this reason that theories will evolve around oral (eating) and anal (defecating) activities: "we can say in general of the sexual theories of children that they are reflections of their own sexual constitution" (Ibid.: 196).[10]

The idea that the child has no knowledge of sexual difference has consequences for the way children's research is organized. The sexual theories of children start from the premise that everyone, including females, is in possession of a genital zone "such as the boy knows from his own body" (Freud 1908a: 215). Now, as we have seen in the previous chapter, the paradigm for infantile sexual pleasure in 1905 is the lips kissing themselves. Also, we have shown that in infantile sexuality there is no natural (or normal) privileged erogenous zone. The 1915 section on sexual research, however, does not take its starting point in these principles. It builds upon the case study of Little Hans and the 1908 essay on the sexual researches of children in which Freud states the following: "[i]t is precisely in what we must regard as the 'normal' sexual constitution that already in childhood the penis is the leading erogenous zone and the chief autoerotic sexual object" (Ibid.: 215). This statement clearly contradicts his previous views on infantile sexuality in which polymorphous perversity implies that there is no privileging of the genital zone over other zones.[11]

Freud is well aware that insights gained from the case study of Little Hans imply a shift from a theory predominantly based on the analysis of female hysteric patients (notably Dora), in whose sexual lives the genital zone is "relatively less prominent," toward a theory based on the analysis of a young male patient with a very lively interest in his own and other people's "widdlers" (Freud 1909a: 106, 109). However, these new insights do connect to some statements in the 1905 *Three Essays*. There Freud had briefly mentioned that the arousal of a child's sexual life "can also come about spontaneously from internal causes," such as the drive for watching, the "curiosity to see other people's genitals," and a "lively interest in the genitals of their playmates" (Freud 1905c: 191, 192). These initial thoughts had remained unelaborated in 1905 since Freud was focusing on the autoerotic nature of the sexual drives. However, the case of Little Hans – to Freud's own surprise – provided him material for further elaborations on the importance of the drive for watching and the curiosity regarding the sexual organs of other persons.

In the case study of Little Hans, Freud argues that the widdler is the organizing element in Hans's first philosophy of life (*Weltanschuung*); it provides him the criterion to make distinctions (between living and lifeless objects) and comparisons (between himself and other living beings). The child's sexual theories are "widdlercentric." Freud's generalizations concerning the role and status of the male genital zone in the sexual theories of children are based on the particular fact that in Little Hans's sexual life his widdler – and not the mouth or anus – is the leading erogenous zone that organizes his sexual theories and philosophy of life. It is this widdlercentrism in the child's sexual inquiries and theories that constitutes an important factor in establishing the primacy of the genital zone. In the 1915 edition, this widdlercentrism is not confined to the theories of boys. According to Freud, little girls will also immediately accept the existence of the penis when discovering that boys have one, and they will also make it their leading erogenous zone, which results in penis envy and the wish to be a boy (Ibid.: 195). The girl's infantile sexual theories are thus also widdlercentric. However, the analysis of the girl's theories is not further pursued – Freud merely mentions it, and then immediately returns to the boy's perspective.[12]

But what about the step toward knowledge of sexual difference? Under what circumstances will the child be able to recognize and accept the inadequacies of its theories and give them up? In 1915 Freud writes that the conviction that all people have penises "is only abandoned after severe internal struggles (the castration complex)" (Ibid.). In line with what Freud had argued in the case of Little Hans, the child will in the end abandon its philosophy of life through further research, investigations, and inquiries after it becomes aware of the fact that its pursuit of the answer to the one riddle ("Where do babies come from?") remains fruitless. The severe inner struggles first of all concern this stubborn defense of the first theories (despite the fact that they remain fruitless). Also, Freud argues, the inner struggles concern the inevitable changes in the relationship with the first significant persons in the child's life. He further writes that the "first step towards taking an independent attitude in the world" and the abandonment of the first theories will also "imply a high degree of alienation" of the child from the persons (i.e., parents and other family members) it could previously trust (Ibid.: 197). In *Three Essays*, Freud does not further elaborate on this "alienation," but elsewhere – notably in his 1909 "Family Romances" – he does.[13] In that short essay, Freud argues that the child's main "task" is to liberate himself or herself from the authority of the parents, the primal caretakers (Freud 1909b: 237). Since, according to Freud, this liberation is motivated by egoistic drives and is an intellectual achievement not informed by knowledge of sexual difference or motivated by the search for sexual pleasure, he characterizes this process of liberation/alienation as "asexual." It is only in puberty that the relations with the parents become "sexualized" (Ibid.: 239). Hence, an "asexual" infantile period is followed by a sexualization that characterizes puberty. We mention this short essay here because despite the apparent absence of a reference to infantile sexuality, the essay is still structured in line with *Three Essays* and the theory of the two regimes of sexuality. Yet the essay also reveals an important motive for the introduction of the notion of a sexual object choice in early childhood and of the Oedipus complex shortly afterward (Freud 1910a; see p. 49),[14] for the thesis of a sexualization of objects in puberty based on knowledge of sexual difference paves the way for the conclusion Jung will draw from such explorations: the infantile period may best be described as "presexual," and infantile sexuality could be considered the result of a phantasmatic reconstruction of childhood in terms of pubertal sexuality (*Zurückphantasieren*) (Haute & Westerink 2020). Freud could only avoid this conclusion and preserve the idea of infantile sexuality by situating what was first considered pubertal (sexual object choice) in the infantile period.

In the 1915 edition, the section on children's sexual research and theories is introduced to map the child's first sexual interest in objects – notably other people's genitals – which in the end inevitably results in the recognition of sexual difference. The infantile research and theories also show, according to Freud, that already in early childhood the male genital zone becomes the leading erogenous zone *in and through the theories* that, as we have said, spring from a riddle that in itself is not sexual. In this way, Freud makes plausible the later primacy of the genitals in adult sexuality.

From hysteria to paraphrenia: narcissism and the problem of the object

In the original edition of *Three Essays*, the change from autoerotic infantile sexuality to objectal adult sexuality does not, according to Freud, imply any special problem. Initially, he seemed to think that this change comes about in most cases on the basis of biological factors and without special difficulties. However, the years prior to and after 1905 also see Freud engaged in an intense correspondence and passionate debate with Jung about psychosis and the drive and libido theory. In 1907 Jung published his book on dementia praecox, in which he stresses the similarities between hysterical symptomatology, mechanisms, and "complexes"[15] on the one hand and dementia praecox on the other. This is instrumental to the reorganization of nosological categories we mentioned in the previous chapter and is at least partially due to a rediagnosing of many hysterical patients as instead suffering from paraphrenia, dementia praecox, paranoia, psychosis, or schizophrenia (a term introduced by Bleuler and used from 1911 onward). In his book Jung also mentions the memoirs of Senatspräsident Schreber for the first time in the history of psychoanalytic thinking (Jung 1907). Freud would return to these famous memoirs in his case study on Schreber, published in 1911, which contains his most well-articulated theory of psychotic pathology (Freud 1911).

The systematic reflection on psychosis that Freud began in his discussions with Jung confronted him with the fact that both the object and the ego that supports our relation to the object have a precarious status. The most central aspect of Schreber's pathology is indeed the conviction of "the imminence of a great catastrophe, of the end of the world" (*Weltuntergangserlebnis*) (Ibid.: 68). At some point Schreber was convinced that this catastrophe had already occurred and that he was the only remaining "real human being." The few people he still saw were nothing but "miracled up, cursorily improvised men" (Ibid.). But in some moments, the opposite tendency broke through. In these moments, Schreber saw his own obituary in the paper and thought that "he himself existed in a second, inferior shape, and in this second shape he one day quietly passed away" (Ibid.). However, the delusion in which the world was destroyed and he was the only remaining human being was by far the strongest. Schreber mentions a list of possible explanations for this catastrophe. He thinks that the earth was frozen because of the withdrawal of the sun, but he also blames his doctor, Flechsig, whose sorcery would have introduced anxiety among people and who would have been at the basis of a destruction of the foundations of religion. This would have caused the spreading of nervousness and immorality, which in turn would have caused the plagues that hit humankind. Similar catastrophes also play a role, according to Freud, in a great number of cases of paranoia. Hence, the "great catastrophe" Schreber is writing about is a defining characteristic of what Freud here calls "paraphrenia."[16] The reference to "miracled up, cursorily improvised men" points the way to a possible explanation of this experience, as this results from an unconscious withdrawal of libidinal ties from both real and phantasmatic objects. The world loses its importance; it becomes indifferent and incoherent. The "miracled up, cursorily improvised men" should be seen as a secondary rationalization in response to this subjective catastrophe: "[t]he end of the world is the projection of this internal catastrophe; his subjective world has come to an end since his withdrawal of his love from it" (Ibid.: 70). It comes as no surprise that, from this perspective, the psychotic delusions have to be interpreted not so much as the product of the disease, but rather as an effort to cure it. The delusion leads the libido back to the persons and things that were first abandoned.

The *Weltuntergangserlebnis* does not exhaust Schreber's delusions. He also believed that he would be transformed into a woman. We do not want to go into all the different aspects and meanings this idea had in the course of Schreber's illness. We simply want to indicate that Schreber thought at some point that this transformation would allow him to be impregnated by God himself. In this way, he would be the origin of a new race of men, and this would allow him to save the world. Schreber's pathology thus exemplifies the delusion of grandeur that characterizes so many psychotic states (Ibid.: 73).

Freud had no choice but to tackle the problem of Schreber's "great catastrophe" and to explain the origin of the delusion of grandeur, if he wanted to broaden the scope of his theories beyond transference neuroses. He had to give these phenomena a place in his developing metapsychology, but at the same time he definitely did not want to give up the primacy of sexuality. The withdrawal from reality that characterizes psychosis clearly was not a problem of the drives for self-preservation. Psychotic patients continue to fulfill their vital needs most of the time. In this perspective, the problematic character of Freud's structural opposition between sexuality and self-preservation, which also structures the first edition of *Three Essays*, once again became obvious. Both Jung and Bleuler argued against Freud that the "loss" of reality that characterizes psychosis cannot be explained in (sexual) libidinal terms. Freud, however, wanted to use the theories he developed to understand hysteria and obsessional neurosis to explain "paraphrenia." He did not think – or did not want to accept – that the psychotic aspects of Schreber's clinical picture would oblige us to give up the elementary distinction between the sexual drive and drives for self-preservation or to rethink his theory of the drives. Since our relation to reality obviously cannot be reduced to his narrow definition of self-preservation – thirst and hunger – Freud had no choice but to consider this relation as essentially sexual if he wanted to maintain his dualistic drive theory that had been the starting point of his 1905 *Three Essays*. The conflicts with Jung over libido theory and with Adler over the nature of the ego in its function of relating to objects (through aggression, power) were born from this commitment.

In his 1912 *Wandlungen und Symbole der Libido*, Jung had explained at great length that psychosis could not be understood in terms of Freud's dualistic drive theory. According to Jung, the withdrawal of objects from reality that characterizes psychosis cannot be understood in sexual terms. This withdrawal has a more general character – it concerns all general psychic interest and involvement in the outside world. As a result, we can only understand psychosis if we redefine the libido as a general psychic interest, of which sexuality is only one of the many possible specifications. For his own argumentation, Jung called upon Freud's 1905 *Three Essays*, notably the first description of the drive as initially being "not itself sexual" and as only becoming sexual through an "organ whose excitation lends the drive a sexual character" (see previous chapter, p. 20). In *Wandlungen*, Jung argues that Freud had suggested here a single primal drive (*Urlibido*) that, in the process of the child's maturation, splits off in various directions (e.g., ambition, thought) and, in connection with certain bodily functions, zones, and objects, becomes cathected with sexuality. In other words, through a process of differentiation, specialization, and maturation of bodily functions during puberty,[17] the primal drive will partly develop into a sexual drive connected to the sexual function of specific body parts (such as the genitals and the lips) that previously (in childhood) had no such function. Hence, whereas Freud thought of the sexual drive as a composition of partial drives, Jung regarded the sexual drive as the effect of the differentiation of the primal libido. He compared this *Urlibido* to Arthur Schopenhauer's will when describing it as "a continuous life impulse, a will to live which will attain the creation of the whole species through the preservation of the individual" (Jung 1912a: 145). This primal libido is thus an instinct for both self-preservation and the preservation of the species. Freud obviously had fundamental problems with this view for several reasons, of which we can here briefly mention only the most important. First, there is Jung's critique of Freud's starting point in *Three Essays*; namely, the distinction between the instinct for nutrition and the sexual drive. Second, there is Jung's rejection of Freud's theory of infantile sexuality as first and foremost the autoerotic experience of pleasure. Instead – and third – Jung favors a functional approach to sexuality, arguing that childhood could best be regarded as a "presexual period" even though one finds in it the germs and first manifestations of a drive (instinct) for the preservation of the species, which, through a process of maturation, will eventually determine adult sexual life, i.e., sexuality in the service of reproduction (Jung 1912b: 126–143). From this we can conclude that while conceptualizing his own depth-psychological theories in a new way, Jung essentially remained faithful to the fundamental premises of the contemporary psychiatrists and sexologists that Freud had severely criticized in the 1905 *Three Essays*.

The problems we are discussing here and the disagreement with Jung on the drive and libido theory constitute the context that compelled Freud to introduce narcissism as a normal phase in psychosexual development (Freud 1905c: 218–219). Freud very explicitly mentions both the withdrawal of the libido from objects and persons and the delusion of grandeur that characterizes "paraphrenia" as an "urgent motive" to introduce the notion of narcissism in his theory (Freud 1914a: 74). More specifically, Freud thought that he needed a theory of narcissism to explain this delusion and withdrawal without giving up the dualistic theory of the drives he had developed in the context of his study of the neuroses (Ibid.: 76–81). Indeed, Freud's theory of narcissism turns the ego into a libidinal construct. This allows Freud to interpret the vicissitudes of this ego that characterize psychosis in libidinal terms and to adapt his old drive theory to the new pathologies he was studying without fundamentally changing it. At least this is Freud's intention. In the next chapter, we will see that the narcissism theory is crucial for understanding later writings in which Freud will fundamentally reconsider his drive theory.

Freud first referred to narcissism in *Three Essays* in a footnote on homosexuality that he added in 1910 (May-Tolzmann 2015a: 21–62). It anticipates the insights into the genesis of a specific kind of homosexuality that Freud developed more extensively in his study on Leonardo da Vinci that was published a few months later (Freud 1910b: 98–100). In the 1910 footnote from *Three Essays*, narcissism is indeed mentioned as one of the possible explanations for what he calls "inversion" (homosexuality): "they proceed from a narcissistic basis, and look for a young man who resembles themselves and whom they may love as their mother loved them" (Freud 1905c: 145). In his 1911 study on Schreber, Freud explicitly links narcissism to psychosis for the first time:

> [t]here comes a time in the development of the individual *at which he unifies his sexual instincts* (which have hitherto been engaged in auto-erotic activities) in order to obtain a love-object; and he begins by taking himself, his own body, as his love-object.
>
> *(Freud 1911: 61, emphasis ours)*

In this perspective, the psychotic withdrawal from reality is interpreted as a regression to these early stages of development in which outside reality did not yet play a role. This regression also explains the psychotic delusions of grandeur: the libidinal cathexis that is withdrawn from the objects is, in the case of psychotic pathology, reinvested in the ego itself. The passage from the study on Schreber anticipates the famous definition of narcissism that we find in "On Narcissism: An Introduction":

> we are bound to suppose that a unity comparable to the ego cannot exist in the individual from the start; the ego has to be developed. The auto-erotic instincts, however, are there from the very first; so there must be something added to auto-erotism – a new psychical action – in order to bring about narcissism.
>
> *(Freud 1914a: 76–77)*

The ego comes into being through the unification of the autoerotic (partial) drives. This unification is intrinsically linked to the choice of one's own body as the first love object of these drives. This unification and this choice are like two sides of the same coin. One cannot be understood apart from the other.

In *Three Essays*, Freud discusses the problem of narcissism in the paragraph on "Libido Theory" that he inserted in the third edition of the text. We find this new paragraph in the chapter "The Transformations of Puberty." It mainly recapitulates positions Freud defended extensively in "On Narcissism" from 1914. In this new paragraph, Freud immediately rejects the Jungian position on the nature of the libido. The libido should be distinguished from "the energy which must be supposed to underlie mental processes in general" (Freud 1905c: 217). Freud does not provide clinical arguments here for the distinction at hand. The latter, he writes, expresses the presumption that "sexual processes" occurring in the organism are distinguished from the nutritive processes by a "special chemistry" (Ibid.). The reference to a "special chemistry" implies that even if it is not possible to clinically distinguish the sexual drives and the drives for self-preservation from the outset, they are always already separated at a more fundamental organic level. This argumentation makes it impossible to understand the sexual libido as an ulterior specification of a primal drive, as Jung proposed (Ibid.: 218).

Freud reminds us in the same context once again that sexual excitation is not derived from the genital parts alone but from all the bodily organs. Sexuality cannot be reduced to genital sexuality. He then writes:

> [w]e thus reach the idea of a quantity of libido, *the mental representation of which we give the name ego-libido*, and whose production, increase or diminution, distribution and displacement should afford us possibilities for explaining the psychosexual phenomena observed.
>
> *(Ibid., emphasis ours)*

Further in this paragraph, Freud identifies ego-libido with narcissistic libido. The narcissistic libidinal cathexis of the ego is "the original state of things" (Ibid.: 218).[18] The theory of narcissism indeed implies that the individual only turns their libido to outside objects in a second moment, after having first invested their own body as a love object. That is why Freud calls the ego resulting from this investment the libido-reservoir, "from which the object-cathexes are sent out and into which they are withdrawn once more" (Ibid.). The ego-libido, Freud writes, only becomes accessible once it is turned into object-libido; that is, only once it is cathexing sexual objects. The vicissitudes of the object-libido become clear from and can be studied in transference neuroses (hysteria and obsessional neuroses).[19] The ego-libido, Freud further writes, plays a major role in the explanation of psychotic disturbances, but as a result of the limitations of the method of psychoanalytic research, we are unfortunately left for the moment to speculation: "[f]rom the vantage-point of psycho-analysis we can look across a frontier, which we may not pass" (Ibid.).[20]

Is the introduction of narcissism in the third edition of *Three Essays* merely an addition to the text or does it also tend to change its fundamental conceptuality? It becomes clear from our explanation that the introduction of narcissism is meant to progressively orient (infantile) sexuality toward the object. Freud thus formulated an alternative to Jung's views on human sexuality as a developmental maturation process characterized by differentiation and functionalization. According to Freud, the ego is the first object of the libido *sexualis*. Narcissism has both a structural aspect – "[it] is merely covered by the later extrusions of the libido, but in essentials remains behind them" (Ibid.) – and a developmental one. Narcissism is a moment on a developmental line that starts with autoerotism and leads to the libidinal investment of outside reality. As a result, infantile sexuality is no longer without an object, as it was before. This is soon confirmed by Freud in "Instincts and Their Vicissitudes," when he argues that although the object is not originally connected with the drive, it becomes assigned to it as a result of being fitted to make satisfaction possible. This object is not necessarily an object in the outside world: "it may equally well be a part of the subject's own body" (Freud 1915: 122).

But there is more. In his study on Schreber, for instance, Freud not only states that the individual first takes their own body as a love object but also adds that the "line of development then leads on to the choice of an external object with similar genitals – that is, to homosexual object choice – and thence to heterosexuality" (Freud 1911: 61). In a passage from 1915, Freud writes:

> [t]he final outcome of sexual development lies in what is known as the normal sexual life of the adult, in which the pursuit of pleasure comes under the sway of the reproductive function and in which the component instincts, under the primacy of a single erogenous zone, form a firm organization directed towards a sexual aim attached to some extraneous sexual object.
>
> *(Freud 1905c: 197)*

This heteronormative developmental approach is intrinsically linked to the introduction of narcissism and will become stronger in the subsequent editions of the text. This is in line with the way Freud introduced the transformations of puberty in the first edition.

Pre-genital organizations and the developmental perspective

The developmental perspective was almost completely absent from the 1905 edition of *Three Essays*. But in the 1915 edition and afterward, Freud thinks that the constitution of the sexual object is the result of a psychic evolution that needs to be studied in great detail and in the course of which many things can go wrong. In this context, Freud also rethinks the status of the erogenous zones in a fundamental way. Whereas in the 1905 edition these zones and the drives of which they are the seats are considered to act anarchically until the primacy of the genital zone is established, Freud now progressively orders them in a temporal sequence. In his "The Disposition to Obsessional Neurosis," published in 1913, Freud introduces the concept of pre-genital organization and describes an anal organization of the libido (Freud 1913). In the 1915 edition of *Three Essays*, he adds a new paragraph on "The Phases of Development of the Sexual Organization" in which he recognizes the existence of an oral, cannibalistic organization of the libido that precedes the anal phase he had described two years earlier (Freud 1905c: 197–200).[21] These pre-genital phases are "abortive beginnings and preliminary stages of a firm organization of the component instincts such as this – preliminary phases which themselves constitute a sexual regime of a sort" (Ibid.: 197–198). These phases are called pre-genital because the genitals do not yet play a dominant role in sexual life. Freud adds that these pre-genital organizations only become active and apparent in pathological cases. This idea clearly strengthens the insight that the different psychopathologies are in fact "abnormal" developmental disturbances. They express problematics that are intrinsically linked to specific developmental phases, such as pre-genital organizations. At first glance, Freud seems to underscore his patho-analytic approach here: the perversions give insight into otherwise smoothly traversed and mostly hidden pre-genital organizations. But on closer inspection, his ideas once again come close to his predecessors: there is "normal" development, and there are "abnormal" disturbances that manifest in perversions.

The first developmental phase is the oral ("cannibalistic") phase. Here, "in this sexual regime," sexuality is not yet distinguished from the ingestion of food. Freud adds that the *object* of both activities is the same. In doing so, Freud is clearly suggesting that sexuality in the oral phase is already directed toward an object. This idea is linked to the fact that the aim of oral sexuality is not merely one of obtaining pleasure at the level of the oral zone ("the lips") but also of *incorporating* the object (Ibid.: 198). This implies that the role of the object is no longer purely instrumental with regard to pleasure, but rather that the drive wants to do something specific ("incorporation") with it. This inevitably contradicts the strong version of autoerotism he had defended in the first edition. What happens to autoerotism in this context? In 1915, Freud considers "blissful sucking":

> a relic of this constructed phase of organisation, which is forced upon our notice by pathology . . . in which the sexual activity, detached from the nutritive activity, has substituted for the extraneous object one situated in the subject's own body.
>
> (*Ibid.*)

Several different points are important here. First, Freud states that no direct observation of the original oral stage of the libido is possible. Certain severe pathological states – which Freud does not specify – oblige us to affirm the existence of such a sexual stage. But this means that thumb-sucking, rather than a *sui generis* activity that can be described for its own sake, now can only be understood as a moment in development from which it receives its meaning.[22] In the first edition, sexuality is said to originate "anaclitically" in the satisfaction of the vital functions of the body. This means that sexuality is identified as the pleasure experienced at the moment of this satisfaction (and, basically, as the excitation caused by the experience of the warm stream of milk). What is at stake here is the pleasure for which the object is instrumental and, hence, the possibility of describing this moment in exclusively physiological terms. In 1915, however, the drive "targets" the object, in a manner of speaking. Pleasure inevitably becomes a secondary effect that accompanies the relation to the object that it wants to make part of itself. The very notion of *Anlehnung* changes its meaning here. It no longer refers to the pleasure found in the experience of vital satisfaction but to the fact *that sexuality originally has the same object as the drive for self-conservation*. Sexuality is no longer about the pleasure caused by the warm milk but about the breast as part of an object that the drive wants to incorporate. The thumb is no longer a part of one's own body that allows one to find pleasure at the level of the oral zone ("the lips") but is now an object that *replaces* the breast. The thumb becomes a substitute, i.e., an *Ersatzobjekt*. This metaphorical process cannot be described in purely physiological terms. It is hard to conceive without the intervention of phantasy. This passage explains why Laplanche can write that sexuality, in the proper sense of the word, comes into being when it *becomes* autoerotic (replaces an outside object with a part of one's own body). He then identifies the drive's becoming autoerotic with sexuality's becoming phantasmatical (Laplanche 1987: 71–72). This contradicts, however, what Freud argues in 1905.

The second pre-genital phase is the anal-sadistic organization. Freud writes that in this organization the polarity that characterizes sexual life – the polarity between "male" and "female" – is already present but only as a polarity between *activity* and *passivity*. Freud immediately links activity to the drive for mastery that unfolds itself through the musculature, which is the organ of the active sexual aim. This illustrates an idea we mentioned previously: in the 1915 edition, the drive for mastery no longer *becomes* sexual through a process of anastomosis, but rather is always already integrated into the sadistic component of the sexual drive.[23] The organ of the passive sexual aim, on the contrary, is primarily the "erotogenic mucous membrane of the anus" (Ibid.). Freud concludes by saying that in this second phase both sexual polarity and the (relation to the) object can be empirically observed.[24]

In *Three Essays*, the oral phase and the anal-sadistic phase are the only pregenital organizations Freud discusses. However, in "The Infantile Genital Organization of the Libido," published in 1923 and explicitly presented as a supplement to *Three Essays*, Freud mentions the existence of a phallic phase that succeeds the two previous ones (Freud 1923a: 142). In the third edition of *Three Essays*, Freud writes the following on the choice of an object:

> [it] has already frequently or habitually been effected during the years of childhood: that is to say, the whole of the sexual currents have become directed towards a single person in relation to whom they seek to achieve their aims. This then is the closest approximation possible in childhood to the final form taken by sexual life after puberty.
>
> *(Freud 1905c: 199)*

However, Freud adds to this passage that in the infantile period the submission of the partial drives to the genitals does not yet occur. This changes in the text from 1923 that we just referred to. Freud now claims that this submission takes place in the infantile period. Freud writes, more particularly, that although there is no real bundling of the partial drives under the primacy of the genital organs during the infantile period, the genitals play a role at the height of the infantile period that is very similar to the one they will later play in adulthood. The main difference between this period and adult sexuality, Freud now says, is the fact that for the little child only the male genital organ plays a (psychological) role. Freud concludes that there "is not a primacy of genitality, but a primacy of the phallus" (Freud 1923a: 142). He introduces these insights in a footnote and in an added sentence in the 1924 edition of *Three Essays* (Freud 1905c: 199, 233).

In the anal-sadistic organization, the sexual difference between "male" and "female" did not yet play a role. This organization only knows the distinction between activity and passivity. The fundamental opposition that characterizes the new phallic organization is between "male genital" and "castrated" (Freud 1923a: 145). The latter will be replaced by the polarity between male and female in the course of puberty. This is the "normal" outcome of psychosexual development that should be understood from the perspective of reproduction. Indeed, Freud understands the oral, anal-sadistic, and phallic organizations from the perspective of their *telos*, which is none other than their submission to and integration into the reproductive function: "[i]n this phase, therefore, sexual polarity and an extraneous object are already observable. But organization and subordination to the reproductive function are still absent" (Freud 1905c: 198–199). From this perspective, Freud is obliged to situate the pre-genital organizations on a developmental line that is directed toward the constitution of a heterosexual object. This was expressed in the Schreber case (see previous discussion), when Freud argued that the "line of development then leads on to the choice of an external object with similar genitals – that is, to homosexual object choice – and thence to heterosexuality" (Freud 1911: 61). The later editions of *Three Essays* are clearly characterized by a strong tendency to reintroduce such heteronormative perspective, which contradicts the critique of the "psychiatric style of reasoning" that is present in the first edition. This tendency implies a reevaluation of the status of homosexuality. Therefore, before proceeding with our discussion of the problem of the object in early childhood, we will first discuss Freud's shifting perspectives on homosexuality.

New perspectives on homosexuality

In the previous chapter, we stated that Freud deals extensively with the issue of homosexuality, arguing that the predominant theories on homosexuality (specific neuropathic disposition, innateness and acquisition, anatomical and psychical hermaphroditism, homosexuality as intermediate stage) fall short with regard to its etiology. Instead, he points at bisexuality as a possible source, not in its crude and banal form of the feminine brain in the masculine body but in the more subtle form he finds in men's love of boys and young adolescents in ancient Greece. What attracted Greek adult men to boys was the combination of the characteristics of both sexes they found in these boys' mental qualities (i.e., virtues such as shyness, modesty, and submissiveness to instruction) and physical appearances – "there is, as it were, a compromise between an impulse that seeks for a man and one that seeks for a woman, while it remains a paramount condition that the object's body (i.e. genitals) shall be masculine" (Freud 1905c: 144).[25] The point Freud wants to draw attention to is this combination of characteristics of both sexes as opposed to the other contemporary theoretical approaches that always start from the premise of sexual differentiation. Yet he also writes that he is not much interested in providing a satisfactory explanation of the origin of homosexuality – and this is understandable given the fact that in 1905 he wants to focus on the autoerotic nature of infantile sexuality. Of greater importance to him is the fact that the analysis of homosexuality leads to a fundamental reconsideration of the relation between the sexual drive, its object, and its aims.

Freud's views on homosexuality change substantially in the period between 1905 and 1915. In general, we can say that he shifts attention from the general connection between bisexuality and homosexuality toward the problem of etiology – infantile object choice – and of the connection between homosexuality and heterosexuality. The 1910 and 1915 footnotes on this issue bear witness to this. The footnote on homosexuality added in 1910 is one of the longer passages inserted in that edition (Ibid.: 144–145, in note). In this footnote, Freud no longer associates homosexuality, as illustrated by ancient Greek men's love of boys and adolescents, as grounded in a bisexual disposition. Instead, the 1910 footnote draws upon his views on homosexuality as depicted in his study of Little Hans and as described in his study of Leonardo da Vinci. In this latter study, Freud interprets the great man's homosexual phantasies and object choices as reminiscences of autoerotic excitations (Freud 1910b: 87). Leonardo's first object choice – his overindulging mother – is aimed at continuation of autoerotic pleasure. Unlike Little Hans's stubborn ignorance about the female genitals, Leonardo's desire to see the genitals of other people and compare them with his own eventually leads to the discovery that women (specifically, his mother) lack a penis. This turns his desire for watching into a nausea that will eventually manifest itself as permanent homosexuality. This nausea is not explained by the discovery of the lack of a penis as such but results from another infantile phantasy about this lack as the result of castration and hence of the idea of the female genitals as a wound.[26] This phantasy is crucial to Leonardo's becoming homosexual. The compulsive longing for men, Freud writes in the 1915 *Three Essays*, can thus be interpreted as a result of the ceaseless flight from women (Freud 1905c: 145, in note). According to his reasoning in the case of Leonardo, a man becomes homosexual to avoid becoming heterosexual; that is, to avoid having sexual relations with women. This is obviously a very different argumentation than the earlier reference to the characteristics of both sexes in bisexuality and to homosexuality as one of many possible modes of sexuality (need for variation). However, the nausea for women is not enough to explain Leonardo's homosexuality, i.e., his attraction to young adults and male students. A second decisive factor is the repression of the love for the mother by identifying with her and taking her position – a position marked by the overindulgence of the mother for her son – and making his own person into the prototype for the choice of love objects. Leonardo has now become a homosexual, says Freud – someone whose love objects are merely substitutional objects of his own childhood person. The objects he now loves are akin to himself being loved by his mother. This is what Freud calls the narcissistic object choice (Freud 1914a: 87–91): "[t]hat is to say, they proceed from a narcissistic basis, and look for a young man who resembles themselves and whom they may love as their mother loved them" (Freud 1905c: 145, in note). The basic characteristic of this type of object choice is the continuation of self-love through object love. We thus find two views of homosexuality (Freud presents them as complementary) in the one 1910 footnote: first, homosexuality as the avoidance of heterosexuality and, second, homosexuality as the outcome of identification with the mother and the continuation of the mother's love.

Yet instead of continuation, Freud in his study of Leonardo speaks of "regression" to a phase of autoerotism. This is a prelude to the next step in Freud's thought on homosexuality and narcissism – a step that eventually leads to yet another reformulation of homosexuality, subsequently added to the same footnote in 1915.[27] To understand the scope of this addition, it is important to briefly consider Freud's case study of Schreber. There he argues that Schreber's apparent homosexuality is to be associated with a stage or phase in the developmental history of the libido (Freud 1911: 61). Narcissism is a stage characterized by the fact that the person brings his autoerotic sexual drives into unity with the aim of choosing one's own body as love object. The first object choice (one's own body) is thus narcissistic, and this choice determines the next developments – namely, first, the homosexual object choice (object with the same body characteristics, i.e., with the same genitals) and, second, the heterosexual object choice in which the genitals are put in the service of procreation and the homosexual impulses are now used for the constitution of social feelings of friendship, comradeship, and love of humankind. Homosexuality is thus no longer primarily seen as a mode of sexuality alongside heterosexuality, in a range of variations regarding the sexual object and aim, but is now seen as a stage in a sexual developmental process that normally tends toward heterosexuality. That means that manifest adult homosexuality can now be opposed to normal sexuality, and this is exactly what can be witnessed in the 1915 footnote. Despite the statement that homosexuals cannot be opposed to or separated from the rest of humankind as a group with a special character (i.e., with a specific neuropathic disposition) because of the fact that all human beings either consciously or unconsciously display homosexual object choices, Freud does make a distinction between the two main "directions" of object choice in terms of "normal" versus "inverted." The latter is associated with the predominance of archaic constitutions and primitive psychical mechanisms, such as narcissistic object choice and "a retention of the erotic significance of the anal zone" (Freud 1905c: 146, in note). In this new predominant perspective (a developmental approach), homosexuality is situated in a heteronormative framework consisting of subsequent phases tending toward a heterosexual object and aim. It is in this context that Freud can refer to homosexuality in terms of regression to an earlier stage.

In the course of this change in perspective, the connection between homosexuality and bisexuality is deconstructed. Freud is explicit about this when he writes:

> [i]t may be insisted that the concept of inversion in respect of the sexual object should be sharply distinguished from that of the occurrence in the subject of a mixture of sexual characters. In the relation between these two factors, too, a certain degree of reciprocal independence is unmistakably present.
>
> *(Ibid.)*

This statement is the direct result of the new approach to homosexuality as a phase originating in the narcissistic object choice. In this context, homosexuality is not seen as avoidance of heterosexuality or as the outcome of identification with the mother. It is the continuation of the love of oneself via an object that embodies what one is, was, or would like to be (Freud 1914a: 88, 90). In this new framework, bisexuality has no longer any substantial role to play.

With regard to homosexuality, not only is there a shift in approach to the subject in the years between 1905 and 1915, but the problematic depiction of homosexuality itself is also puzzling. In the 1905 *Three Essays* and the Leonardo study, Freud associates homosexuality with the attraction to boys, adolescents, young men, and male students. In the Schreber case, Freud has no problem identifying Schreber's transgender wish to become a woman through removal of the male genitals, without any fear of castration (and hence not troubled by inherited schemes or complexes), as homosexuality. But surely transsexuality and homosexuality are not the same (Vandermeersch 2017). By giving homosexuality a place in a developmental scheme, Freud does not provide satisfying answers to the question of what homosexuality is or what forms of it one might want to distinguish. We could perhaps conclude from this fact that Freud is not really interested in developing a coherent conceptualization of homosexuality (Dean 2001) but is instead interested in the more fundamental question of the relation between infantile sexuality and later object finding. And this is indeed the fundamental question that had remained a riddle in the 1905 theory of sexuality.

The diphasic introduction of the object

It is clear that Freud's theory of the pre-genital organizations, as he introduced them in the third edition of *Three Essays*, breaks in a very essential way with the perspective of autoerotic infantile sexuality that characterized the 1905 edition. In the first edition, the developmental perspective was hardly present, and Freud mentions only two "phases" in the development of the infant: infantile masturbation and its return at the age of three (Freud 1905a: 48–49). In the 1915 edition, however, Freud claims that the object is installed in two phases:

> [i]t may be regarded as typical of the choice of an object that the process is diphasic, that is, that it occurs in two waves. The first of these begins between the age of two and five and is brought to a halt or to a retreat by the latency period; it is characterized by the infantile nature of the sexual aims. The second wave sets in with puberty and determines the final outcome of sexual life.
>
> *(Freud 1905c: 200)*

This diphasic structure is mainly due, according to Freud, to the repression that occurs in the latency period.[28] It is important to note that what is repressed here are not oral or anal pleasures, as was the case in Freud's first theory of sexuality, but rather specific objects that are forbidden (e.g., the parents). This shows once again that Freud in the later editions of his text considers the infantile period as very similar to the adult one. Freud further writes that the object choices from the infantile period can have lasting effects. Their sexual aims become mitigated and are at the basis of what Freud calls the "affective current" of sexual life.

We mentioned the problematic status of tenderness in the first edition of *Three Essays*,[29] wherein Freud wrote that *during the period of latency* the child learns to love other people who assist it in its helplessness and satisfy its needs. And as we know already, Freud further specifies that it is "a love on the model and in continuation of the relationship of the infant to its nursing caregiver" (Freud 1905a: 73). Freud reduces tenderness to inhibited sexuality in this context for the reasons we previously discussed. The tender relations to the caregivers that are established during the latency period are forms of inhibited sexuality. These caregivers – in particular the parents – then become the first (phantasmatic) objects of the sexual libido at the beginning of puberty. However, the incest barrier forces the child to choose other objects for his or her libido. We explained why this theory of tenderness from the first edition is at odds with the idea that infantile sexuality is essentially autoerotic, which Freud defends at the same time. Indeed, how can the child's love for the caregiver(s) be understood as a form of inhibited sexuality if one turns to the object only at the beginning of puberty? The diphasic introduction of the object seems to solve this problem because it implies that the sexual libido already invests in a number of objects (persons) before the latency period. The libidinal investment of these objects is repressed at the beginning of the latency period and what remains is a tender relationship toward these objects.

Most readers will have thought of the Oedipus complex while reading the previous paragraphs. It is indeed fair to say that the third edition of *Three Essays* prepares the introduction of this famous complex, which was, as we already know, literally unthinkable, at least in its canonical form,[30] in the editions from 1905 and 1910. As long as Freud considered infantile sexuality to be essentially non-objectal, oedipal problems belonged to puberty. This changes when infantile sexuality is thought to have an object from the outset and when its introduction is said to have a diphasic character. All the conditions are now put in place to further concretize the relation of the little child to the object and to itself from the perspective of the infantile relation to the *parental* objects. The lasting effects of the first object choices Freud talks about then become identical to the lasting psychological effects of the libidinal relations toward the parents.

All of this reminds us of the theory of the Oedipus complex that belongs to the phallic phase of psychosexual development (Freud 1923a). It is indeed in this phase that the little child can relate to a single person while its partial drives are already subsumed under the primacy of the genital organs. However, the Oedipus complex is hardly mentioned in *Three Essays*. It is only discussed in two footnotes that were added to the text in 1920 (Freud 1905c: 162, 226). What explains this absence in the later editions of *Three Essays*? This is an important question because our efforts to answer it will confront us with crucial concepts that are lacking in Freud's theory of sexuality of both 1905 and 1915. Without these crucial concepts – one can think, for instance, of identification and the superego function – the Oedipus complex cannot be properly articulated. We will thematize this problem in our next chapter, but first we will discuss two elements that seem peripheral to Freud's theory of sexuality but in fact will be crucial to understanding the meaning of our text in the Freudian corpus.

The role of chemical substances

The fact that Freud largely described sexuality (pleasure) in 1905 in terms of physiological processes, i.e., the excitability of erogenous zones, had implications for his perspective on some fundamental questions concerning, first, the question of the origin and nature of sexual pleasure and unpleasure and, second, the question of how and why sexual pleasure could be accompanied by sexual tension if one begins from the premise that pleasure equals tension reduction (Ibid.: 209). Freud had already raised these questions in 1896, arguing that unpleasure could not result from external forces – restrictive cultural conventions – and hence had to originate from an as yet unknown "independent" inner source (Freud 1896a: 221–222). In the 1905 edition, Freud comments on this issue that "everything relating to the problem of pleasure and unpleasure touches upon one of the sorest spots of present-day psychology" (Freud 1905c: 209). But since these questions and problems concern the very essence of sexuality, one might at least expect Freud to expand on the physiological processes involved. Indeed, in the 1905 edition, we find Freud addressing the question of the role played by the sexual substances, the internal sexual organs, and the sex glands (Freud 1905a: 69–70). The fact that the 1905 section on the role of the sex gland was replaced in 1920 by a section highlighting the role of the so-called puberty gland (Freud 1905c: 215–216) indicates that theories on these physiological processes were still in flux and that Freud found a convincing theory on the glands that connected well to his own insights only relatively late. It provided not only an answer to the question of the origin of sexual excitation in the earliest stages of life but also a theory that matched well with Freud's views on the phasic development of the sexual characters – a development that Freud is eager to associate with the diphasic model he introduced in 1915 describing the importance of the two periods (the age of 3–5, puberty) that stand out in the formation of a person's sexual life. Let us have a closer look.

A large section in the third essay of the 1905 edition of *Three Essays* is devoted to "the problem of sexual excitation." In this section, Freud states that "we remain in complete ignorance both of the origin and of the nature of the sexual tension which arises simultaneously with the pleasure when erotogenic zones are satisfied" (Ibid.: 212). As a seemingly plausible explanation, he mentions pleasure itself as a source of sexual tension but finds this thesis untenable since the "greatest pleasure of all" – namely, the pleasure that accompanies the discharge of sexual products (ejaculation) – is accompanied by the removal of all tension. Another explanation – Freud mentions Krafft-Ebing in this context – is possibly found in the thesis that "the accumulation of the sexual substances creates and maintains sexual tension" (Freud 1905c: 213). According to Freud, this thesis was designed to account for sexual tension in the lives of adult males and runs counter to the fact that sexual tension can also be found in infantile life, females, and castrated males, i.e., persons who have little or no production of sexual products. Observations of castrated males confirm this, says Freud. The castration – the removal of the sex glands (testicles) – has no effect on the libido, which indicates no causal relation between the function of these glands and sexual tension. Hence, Freud concludes, "we are in the dark as to the organ or organs to which sexuality [*Geschlechtlichkeit*] is attached" (Ibid.: 216).

In 1905, Freud therefore formulates a provisional hypothesis in a subsection called "Chemical Theory" to fill in the gap of knowledge: it is likely that the stimulation of erogenous zones, and hence the onset of sexual excitation, triggers the thyroid gland to produce a substance that is disseminated throughout the whole body. The subsequent decomposition of this substance acts – in manners comparable to a toxic substance – as a stimulus upon the reproductive organs. Freud adds that he attaches no importance to this thesis "and should be ready to abandon it at once in favor of another" (Ibid.). In the 1920 edition, this section on chemical theory is deleted and replaced by a new one, as we have already mentioned. In this new text, Freud states that the recent experimental research on the removal of the sex glands of animals has shed new light on the origin of sexual excitation. The research found that the removal of the testicles or ovaries had a strong effect on the sex of the subjects: the transformation of males into females and vice versa. This transformation was not to be attributed to the parts of the sex glands that produce the sexual products (semen and ova) but to the part identified as the "puberty gland."[31] Freud now assumes that the chemical substances released by the puberty gland into the blood not only produce sexual excitation in the nervous system, and particularly the sexual organs, but also have an effect on primary and secondary male and female sexual characteristics.

In a footnote added in 1920, Freud further explores the role of the puberty gland in the development of sexual characteristics. He quotes from a book on the subject written in 1919 by Alexander Lipschütz, who had argued that the maturation of sexual characteristics in puberty is only an acceleration of a process that begins much earlier in time; namely, during intrauterine life. What had always been called puberty was thus probably only a second major phase of puberty. The period of childhood that lies between birth and this second phase of puberty could then be called "the intermediate phase of puberty." This theory of the maturation of sexual characteristics in two phases is to a certain extent in agreement with psychoanalytic findings, says Freud. The major distinction lies in the fact that psychoanalysis identifies an early efflorescence in infantile sexual life in the period between three and five years old (Ibid.: 177). The advantage of this theory of the puberty gland is that it supports the idea of diphasic sexual development.

The problem of the relation between pleasure and unpleasure continues to remain a sore spot in the later editions of *Three Essays*. In a footnote from 1924,

Freud remarks that it was only first in "The Economic Problem of Masochism" that he was able to make "an attempt at solving this problem" (Ibid.: 209, in note). An attempt indeed, because according to Freud, the fact that the phenomenon of sexual excitation shows that pleasure can be accompanied by increased sexual tension merely means that pleasure and unpleasure cannot depend on the quantitative factor of increased or decreased sexual tension. Freud concludes from this that additional qualitative factors will probably be decisive, adding that this is as yet unexplored territory.[32] Also, the eventual "solution" brought to the fore in the 1924 text on masochism depends heavily on the notions of the death and life drives. For reasons we will explore in the next chapter, Freud chose not to include in *Three Essays* a discussion on the question of the physiological and psychological laws governing the relation between the pleasure-unpleasure principle and the death and life drives.

The historical acquisitions of humankind

Another issue that is seemingly peripheral but in fact touches on central aspects of the theory of sexuality concerns the inheritance of psychic disposition (phylogenesis). With the introduction of the phylogenetically inherited schemata in the 1915 edition, Freud clearly moves away from the model of hysteria dominating the 1905 edition. We will examine this in more detail.

We have seen that in 1905 Freud had questioned the status of accidental events and influences in the etiology of the psychoneuroses. This implied that constitutional and hereditary factors could gain the upper hand. But contrary to his predecessors, Freud did not relate these latter factors to a specific abnormal neuropathic disposition. Instead, he wrote that the polymorphous perverse nature of infantile sexuality in fact described the general human sexual constitution. And he had stressed the organically determined processes in the first structuring of sexuality: drives, erogenous zones, muscular activity, and reaction formations. Concerning the relation between disposition and culture, Freud had argued that cultural morality connects to the first, organically determined psychic patterns that are also "fixed by heredity," and that cultural morality consequently develops organic processes further by adding to them specific culturally determined contents as to what exactly is considered, for example, disgusting or shameful (Ibid.: 177). Freud had merely mentioned that these hereditary factors were "less well known," difficult to investigate, and generally overestimated in their etiological significance by his predecessors in psychiatry and sexology (Ibid.: 173, 236). However, in the preface to the 1915 edition, Freud takes a new perspective on the issue of constitution. He writes that "the phylogenetic disposition can be seen at work behind the ontogenetic process." Or, in other words, "disposition is ultimately the precipitate of earlier experience of the species to which the more recent experience of the individual, as the sum of all accidental factors, is super-added" (Ibid.: 131). Freud therefore shifts attention from a general human polymorphous perverse sexual disposition to the general human disposition as the sum of historical experiences inscribed in the organism. The questions now are how, why, and with what consequences is a theory of inherited phylogenetic material and schemata introduced in the 1915 edition.

The first indication that Freud is considering historical material relevant for the theory of sexuality is already found in the 1910 edition. In a footnote, Freud remarks that the erotic life of antiquity and of the contemporary period differs – in the former the drive is stressed, and in the latter the object is stressed (Ibid.: 149). This remark connects to earlier ideas concerning the influence of historical processes and different "cultural epochs of civilization" on mental life, notably the "advance of repression in the emotional life of mankind."[33] In other words, Freud had already hinted at the relevance of different cultural epochs and contexts within a general evolutionary – or developmental – view of human cultural life, from primitive to advanced societies, before *Three Essays* was written.[34]

Yet only from 1911 onward did Freud begin systematically devoting himself to the study of the origins of culture and religion, morality, and social organizations. It is in this context that the question of the acquisition of prehistorical material throughout human history is raised. On the question of how prehistoric experiences can have an impact on later generations, Freud writes that "a part of the problem seems to be met by the inheritance of psychical dispositions which, however, need to be given some sort of impetus in the life of the individual before they can be roused into actual operation" (Freud 1912–1913: 158).[35] The idea that dispositions can only become effective through an accidental factor is not new: we already find this in the Dora case study (Haute 2018). But in the 1915 edition of *Three Essays*, Freud finds it necessary to emphasize this point: "the constitutional factor must await experiences before it can make itself felt; the accidental factor must have a constitutional basis in order to come into operation" (Freud 1905c: 239). The reason for emphasizing this point is linked to the debate with Jung concerning the role of phylogenetic material. Freud wants to avoid a Jungian perspective and therefore dismisses the idea that this material operates in individual life as an autonomous force predetermining individual experiences. If this were the case, psychoanalysis would again be identified with a biological deterministic and teleological view of mental life.

But why and how exactly is the phylogenetic factor in infantile sexuality introduced in the 1915 edition? On this, Freud writes the following:

> [t]he order in which the various instinctual impulses come into activity seems to be phylogenetically determined; so, too, does the length of time during which they are able to manifest themselves before they succumb to the effects of some freshly emerging instinctual impulse or to some typical repression.
>
> *(Ibid.: 241)*

This passage gives us a clear indication as to why and how Freud elaborated the topic of phylogenesis in the 1915 edition. As we have seen previously, in this edition Freud introduced a strong developmental approach, identifying the various phases that are placed in an order generally considered human. The reference to phylogenesis serves to strengthen the claim that the sequence of phases can indeed be presented in a certain order – as Freud does – despite the fact that, according to Freud, in individual cases there seem to occur variations in this temporal sequence and duration. Such individual variations are not random expressions of a "need for variation," for example, as Freud might have said in 1905, but rather deviations of an order that in principle is predetermined.

A first implication of Freud's 1915 line of reasoning is that the relation between cultural morality and organically determined reaction formations becomes more complicated. Whereas in 1905 Freud stressed that culturally morality connects to already established psychic patterns and dams, in 1915 these reaction formations are seen as founded on historical experiences. In a footnote on reaction formations, he writes: "[t]hese forces which act like dams upon sexual development – disgust, shame and morality – must also be regarded as historical precipitates of the external inhibitions to which the sexual drive has been subjected during the psychogenesis of the human race" (Ibid.: 162).[36] Consequently, Freud can no longer think of the origin of repression without reference to the historical experiences of humankind. In the first chapter, we said that cultural morality follows organic processes, but now Freud adds that these organic processes are at least partly following cultural-historical patterns.

But there is more to say about the inheritance of psychic dispositions. In the case study of the Wolf Man, composed in 1914 but first published in 1918, Freud points out that this acquired phylogenetic material includes fear of castration, seduction, and the curiosity and sensibility for (watching or overhearing) parental intercourse (Freud 1918: 97).[37] For example, the Wolf Man immediately and instinctively "knows" the difference between the male and female genitals, just as animals have certain instinctual knowledge of sexual difference and the use of the genital organs.[38] In this case, Freud found clinical evidence for his theories first articulated in *Totem and Taboo*: there are phylogenetically inherited schemata and "complexes" – notably the Oedipus complex – that, like Immanuel Kant's transcendental categories, organize experiences and sometimes even triumph over individual experiences.

> We are often able to see the schema triumphing over the experience of the individual; as when in our present case the boy's father became the castrator and the menace of his infantile sexuality in spite of what was in other respects an inverted Oedipus complex.
>
> *(Ibid.: 119)*

On the level of the experience, the little Wolf Man identified with his mother taking his father as love object – an inverted constellation in which one would expect the mother to now be in the role of castrator. On this point, however, Freud argues that the actual experience is eclipsed by the experiences of the previous generations, for whom the father was the castrator (Marder 2015).

In the case of the Wolf Man, Freud indeed writes of an "instinctive knowledge" that has its analogy in the instinctual "knowledge" of animals. John Fletcher has drawn attention to the fact that Freud uses the word *instinktiv* and not *triebhaft*, which in Fletcher's view tells us that Freud did not view the sexual drive, but rather the underlying phylogenetic schemata and complexes, as analogous to animal instincts. Although the drive may be contingent and variable, it is the phylogenetic schemata that – analogous to instincts – predetermine knowledge, experiences, and reactions to certain impressions and stimuli. But does this mean that Freud is interested in making a clear and well-defined distinction between drive and instinct? We should note that Freud's thought on this matter can hardly be called systematic or consistent. In other writings, for example, we find passages that suggest that the sexual drive is found in both human beings and higher animals.[39] The fact is that in the 1915 edition of *Three Essays*, Freud does not refer to the animal instincts and does not address the topic of the distinction between drive and instinct in the context of the new paragraphs on the phylogenetically inherited material. In *Three Essays*, this distinction seems not to be a topic that concerns Freud (Haute, Kistner & Westerink 2017).

Since these inherited "schemata" and "complexes" include predetermined responses to objects, this theory has an impact on the relation between infantile sexuality and the later transformations in puberty. In the previous chapter, we discussed the issue of trauma, the child's confrontation with adult sexuality at an age at which it is not physiologically and psychologically ready for this encounter, and the reactivation of the memories of such an encounter (or encounters) afterward (*Nachträglichkeit*) in puberty; that is, at an age when the person has gained knowledge of sexual difference and the function of sexual organs. It is only in puberty that a person, now informed about adult sexuality and able to build associations and phantasies around sexual representations, can have a different understanding of what was remembered. With the introduction of the phylogenetic schemata and complexes in 1915, this later understanding of memories from childhood is reinterpreted in terms of a reproduction of experiences that already in childhood are understood – at least to a certain extent – within the context of the inherited schemata and complexes (Fletcher 2013: 69ff, 268–269). Already in early infancy, there is certain inherited knowledge of and phantasies about object-related sexuality.

With the introduction of the phylogenetically inherited schemata in the 1915 edition, we might expect Freud to further elaborate in more detail the content and consequences of the inherited schemata. Yet in the 1915 elaborations on phylogenesis, he does not refer explicitly to the Wolf Man case and the analysis of elements that enter infantile sexual life through the inherited phylogenetic schemata and complexes: the curiosity for genitals and parental intercourse, the fear of castration, the problem of guilt, and of course the Oedipus complex (including ambivalence of feelings and identification). Instead, with regard to phylogenesis, he merely refers to the relevance of this theory for his thoughts on the *order* of developmental phases. And the inherited material listed in the Wolf Man case is mentioned only in the 1920 edition elsewhere in the text; namely, in a footnote where he links these elements to the content of sexual phantasies in puberty. Freud writes:

> [s]ome among the sexual phantasies of the pubertal period are especially prominent, and are distinguished by their very occurrence and by being to a great extent independent of individual experience. Such are the adolescent's phantasies of overhearing his parents in sexual intercourse, of having been seduced at an early age by someone he loves and of having been threatened with castration [. . .] such, too, are his phantasies of being in the womb, and even of experiences there, and the so-called "Family Romance," in which he reacts to the difference between his attitude towards his parents now and in his childhood.
>
> *(Freud 1905c: 226, in note)*

Conclusion

The editions of *Three Essays* from 1915 and later contain a theory of sexuality that is in many respects at odds with the positions Freud defended in 1905. The 1905 edition described a universal (biological) disposition that is at the basis of hysteria in particular and psychopathology in general. This disposition was not primarily understood from a developmental perspective. As a result, psychopathology had a structural and universal meaning. Nobody really escapes pathology. What we call psychopathology is nothing other than the magnification of what is typically human. All of this changes considerably in the later editions. The many additions turn *Three Essays* into a theory of psychosexual development. In this perspective, psychopathology tends to be no longer understood as a structural part of human existence, but rather as a developmental disorder that at least in principle can be avoided. Freud henceforth tends to interpret pathological states as developmental disturbances that are linked to specific pre-genital organizations. According to Freud, these pre-genital organizations are founded in the evolution of humankind. This explains the growing importance of phylogenetic speculation in Freud's thinking. We previously mentioned the letter to Fliess in which Freud added to the announcement of the abandonment of the seduction theory: "the factor of a hereditary disposition regains a sphere of influence from which I had made it my task to dislodge it" (Freud 1985: 265). One could say that in the later editions Freud also remains fundamentally faithful to what he wrote to Fliess in 1897. But one would have to add that the reference to an organic hysterical disposition is fundamentally different from a reference to a phylogenetically determined psychosexual development. All of this implies that in the later editions of *Three Essays*, Freud introduces the idea of what Moll would have called the "principle of teleology," a normal psychological development that at least in principle finds its completion in a heterosexual relation. What began in *Three Essays* as a radical critique of the "popular opinion" on sexuality in this way threatens to become a subtle defense of it (Haute 2002).

The introduction of the Oedipus complex is a crucial element in this shift toward a new psychoanalytic defense of the "popular opinion." Strangely enough, the Oedipus complex is only mentioned twice in the later editions and exclusively in footnotes. We find the most complete version – the "canonical form" – of the Oedipus complex in *The Ego and the Id* from 1923. Hence, it would have been possible for Freud to add a new paragraph on this topic in the last edition of his text (1924), just as he had done with other new and fundamental findings in the previous editions. It is not immediately clear why Freud did not judge it fit to do this. Maybe he realized that developing the meaning and function of the Oedipus complex in great detail might have made it all too obvious that he was progressively reintroducing a conceptuality that radically contradicted the one that determined the outline of the first version. Or maybe he realized that the full articulation of this complex presupposed the introduction of a number of fundamental concepts (such as identification and the superego function) that were not yet mentioned in *Three Essays* and that, more importantly, should not self-evidently be part of a theory of sexuality. Perhaps Freud thought it prudent to refer to the Oedipus complex only in footnotes because he understood that he would otherwise have to rewrite large parts of his text. In the next chapter, we will deal with this question in more detail.

In 1920 Freud published *Beyond the Pleasure Principle*, in which he developed a new theory of the drives. In this text, the opposition between a sexual drive and a drive for self-preservation that had hitherto dominated Freud's thinking is replaced by an opposition between death drives and life drives. Freud hardly mentions this new drive theory in *Three Essays*. He refers to *Beyond the Pleasure Principle* and related texts only indirectly and incidentally when he mentions the problem of erogenous masochism and the problem of sexual tension (Freud 1905c: 158, in note; 168, in note). Here again one could ask why Freud did not attempt to integrate at least partially this crucial development into the last edition of *Three Essays*, just as he had done with other theoretical developments, notably in the 1915 edition. When we try to understand the absence of the Oedipus complex and the new drive theory in the 1920 and 1924 editions of *Three Essays*, we are inevitably faced with the ultimate limitations of the model that was at the basis of Freud's theory of sexuality in this text. In other words, this question will inevitably lead us "beyond" *Three Essays on the Theory of Sexuality*.

Notes

1 In the 1910 *Five Lectures on Psycho-Analysis*, Freud not only introduces the concept of the Oedipus complex and provides a first description of it but also tries to conceptualize the relation between this complex and children's sexual theories given that both, according to Freud, take place in the same period of infantile life (Freud 1910a: 47–48). His comments on this relation between the complex and infantile theories, however, reveal some problems, most importantly the fact that the Oedipus complex presupposes at least certain insight into sexual difference (more specifically, the difference between father and mother), whereas the infantile theories are built on the idea that there is no knowledge of sexual difference (more specifically, the idea that both fathers and mothers have male genitals). Freud does not further explore this issue. It seems significant, though,

that the introduction of the Oedipus complex coincides with a decline of interest in the topic of the *Wißtrieb* and children's sexual theories after the initial texts of 1908/1909. In fact, the 1915 edition of *Three Essays* is the last text in which Freud elaborates this train of thought on infantile sexual theories and the child's lack of knowledge of sexual difference. By that time, Freud had already found in his analyses of the Wolf Man that the child at a very early stage may have knowledge of sexual difference. For further discussion of this issue, see the upcoming section on the phylogenetic factor in infantile sexuality.

2 Compare: "[o]riginally, as we know, the accent was on a portrayal of the fundamental difference between the sexual life of children and of adults; later, the pre-genital organizations of the libido made their way into the foreground, and also the remarkable and momentous fact of the diphasic onset of sexual development. Finally, our interest was engaged by the sexual researches of children; and from this we were able to recognize the far-reaching approximation of the final outcome of sexuality in childhood (in about the fifth year) to the definitive form taken by it in the adult" (Freud 1923a: 141).

3 However, there is some ambiguity on this topic since Freud also mentions that pain could be pleasurable, and he writes that ever since Rousseau we know that the buttocks is one "of the erogenous roots of the passive drive to cruelty" (Freud 1905a: 53). From this perspective, it might make sense to make an equivalence between the reaction formations and pain.

4 This implies that masochism cannot be "primary," as Freud thought in his later years, but is a phenomenon that can only occur at the onset of puberty once sexuality has found its object.

5 Further in the text Freud says once again that the "active" perversion is *regularly* linked to the passive one (Ibid.: 28).

6 We will return to this issue of identification in the next chapter.

7 We will discuss the anal-sadistic organization and the pre-genital organizations later in this chapter.

8 Krafft-Ebing's analyses of fetishism in his *Psychopathia Sexualis* heavily draw upon Binet's view of fetishism as originating from an optical impression accompanied by sexual excitement and taking place in the period of the awakening of the *Vita sexualis* (Krafft-Ebing 1886: 143–146).

9 The "existence of two sexes does not to begin with arouse any difficulties or doubts in children" (Freud 1905c: 195).

10 In a footnote added in 1920, Freud returns to the issue of infantile sexual research and investigations, arguing that the later sexual phantasies, as they appear in puberty, build on the material of these earlier researches and theories; that is to say, on the perverse – oral and anal – components that meanwhile have been repressed (Freud 1905c: 226).

11 One could also think here of Rudolf Reitler's critique on the following passage that we find in the 1905 and 1910 editions of *Three Essays*: "[i]f we survey the sum of these procedures, and consider that soiling something is bound to be similar in its effects to measures for keeping it clean, it is difficult to overlook *nature's purpose*: to establish, through early infantile masturbation (which scarcely a single individual escapes), the future primacy of these erogenous zones for genital activity" (Freud 1905a: 48, emphasis ours). Reitler criticized the teleological nature of this argument in favor of the universality of masturbation. Freud admitted the problematic and changed the phrasing accordingly in the following editions.

12 In the 1920 edition, Freud adds a footnote arguing that the little girl develops not only penis envy when viewing a boy's genitals but also – like boys – an infantile theory in which girls originally had a penis that was lost through castration (Freud 1905c: 195).

13 On the issue of alienation (*Entfremdung*) as redefining one's position in the family romance, see Westerink (2014).

14 "Family Romances" was written shortly before Christmas 1908. The lectures in which Freud introduces the Oedipus complex were held in September 1909 at Clark University.

15 Freud's use of the term *complex* (e.g., castration complex, Oedipus complex) is derived from Jung's terminology as displayed in his 1907 *Über die Psychologie der Dementia Praecox*. Jung introduced this concept in psychiatric literature after the neurologist Theodor Ziehen had first used this concept (in 1898) to define "emotionally charged groups of associations." From this we can understand why we do not find Freud using the term before 1907 (Vandermeersch 1991: 45–48). In "On the History of the Psycho-analytic Movement," Freud himself explicitly mentions the fact that the term *complex* was introduced in psychoanalytic theory by Jung (Freud 1914b: 29–30).

16 Vandermeersch has convincingly argued that the debate (including severe misunderstandings) between Freud and Jung cannot be fully understood if one does not take into account the different models for the reorganization of nosological categories in the contemporary literature. Whereas Kraepelin introduced a distinction between dementia praecox and paranoia – which Jung follows – and Bleuler introduced the term *schizophrenia* in 1911, Freud maintains the use of the older and broader concepts of paraphrenia and paranoia in his Schreber case study and in his 1914 text on narcissism (Vandermeersch 1991: 115–128); see also Freud (1911: 75–76). Freud does not want to follow Kraepelin or Bleuler in their use of the terms *dementia praecox* and *schizophrenia* since both categories had been introduced to create a distinction with what had previously been termed *paranoia*. To avoid this separation, Freud proposes to use the term *paraphrenia*, which has "no special connotation, and it would serve to indicate a relationship with paranoia." The aim of this proposition is that Freud wants to maintain a continuum between the neuroses, paranoia, and the psychoses to claim the extension of psychoanalysis to the realm of the psychoses (Freud 1911: 75–78; Woods 2011: 80–81).

17 According to Jung, "[W]e see the libido at the stage of childhood almost wholly [*zunächst ganz*] occupied in the instinct of nutrition, which takes care of the upbuilding of the body" (Jung 1912a: 148).

18 This reference to an "original state of things" does not imply that Freud identifies autoerotism and narcissism here. This original state is in fact "realized in earliest childhood," meaning that it emerged through a "new psychic action."

19 From 1913 onward, Freud makes a distinction between transference neuroses (hysteria, obsessional neurosis), narcissistic neuroses (dementia praecox, paranoia, melancholia), and actual neuroses (anxiety neurosis, hypochondria). The term *transference neuroses* refers to the psychoanalytic practice and the patient's production of phantasies and impulses in the "transference" relation with the analyst (Freud 1914c: 154).

20 In a 1924 footnote, Freud adds that the analyses of "neuroses other than the transference neuroses" – that is, other than hysteria and obsessional neuroses – have become accessible to psychoanalysis and produced more insight into the relation between narcissism and object-libido. Freud is referring here in particular to the study of melancholia. This will be further discussed in the next chapter.

21 In a series of footnotes in the section on the phases of development of the sexual organization, Freud credits Karl Abraham's contributions to this part of the theory. Indeed, in the period from 1915 to 1924, Abraham will publish several texts on the developmental phases, introducing some new elements, such as an oral-sadistic phase. On this issue, see May Tolzmann (2015a: 127–154).

22 In a footnote to the paragraph on "the finding of an object" that was also added in 1915, Freud refers to the distinction between an anaclitic and a narcissistic type of object choice that he had thematized at great length in "On Narcissism" (Freud 1905c: 222, 1914a: 87–91). The latter refers to those cases in which the individual's object choice is narcissistically motivated. In such cases a person takes a love object that resembles her or him.

23 In the background of this development stands Freud's debate with Adler, who had further developed Freud's notion of the drive for mastery by arguing that through a process

he called *Triebverschränkung* the drive for mastery could become an aspect of all drives. Freud interpreted Adler as introducing a "third drive" alongside the sexual drive and the drive of self-preservation. It is in response to this that Freud, in his case study of Little Hans, chooses not to defend a need for mastery independent of sexual drives, but instead reasons that each drive has "its own power of becoming aggressive" and hence that Hans's hostility toward his father and sadistic impulses toward his mother should be seen as "components of the sexual libido" (Freud 1909a: 141). See also Adler (1908).

24 Freud further associates these aspects of the sadistic-anal organization with the concept of ambivalence – a concept introduced by Bleuler in 1910 in the context of his studies on schizophrenia. In *Three Essays*, Freud seems to give it a different, broader meaning: the appearance of "opposing pairs of drives" (Freud 1905c: 199). In the years preceding the 1915 edition, the concept of ambivalence had already found its way into Freud's writing, mostly describing the contrasting feelings of love and hatred toward significant other persons (parents, loved ones, authorities). See, for example, the second essay of *Totem and Taboo* (Freud 1912–1913: 29, 68).

25 In 1915 Freud underscores this reference to bisexuality by adding that "the sexual object is a kind of reflection of the subject's own bisexual nature" (Freud 1905c: 144).

26 In the case of Leonardo, Freud does not link the phantasy about the female penis (and subsequent castration) to a lack of knowledge of sexual difference but sees it as originating from inherited cultural material.

27 In 1915 Freud deletes a few sentences from the 1910 footnote in which he nuances his statements on homosexuality, arguing that the problem of inversion is highly complex and that there are different types of inversion (Freud 1905c: 145).

28 In the 1920 edition, Freud writes that the diphasic sexual development as well as the interruption by the period of latency "appears to be one of the necessary conditions of the aptitude of men for developing a higher civilization, but also of their tendency to neurosis." This diphasic development, Freud adds, has no analogy in animal life (Freud 1905c: 234).

29 See previous chapter, p. 29.

30 We have already discussed the absence of the Oedipus complex in the previous chapter. We will discuss the absence of this complex in its "canonical form" at length in the next chapter.

31 According to Freud, the puberty gland is likely to have a "hermaphrodite disposition," meaning that it would give anatomical foundation to the theory of bisexuality. In a footnote added in 1920 in the context of the discussion of the homosexual's aim, Freud writes that for this reason recent experiments with the transformation of sex do not justify the idea that homosexuality, for example, is a physiological defect (lack of produced male substance by the glands) that can and should be "cured" through a transplant of testicles (Freud 1905c: 147).

32 Compare: "[i]f we were able to say what this qualitative characteristic is, we should be much further advanced in psychology. Perhaps it is the rhythm, the temporal sequence of changes, rises and falls in the quantity of stimulus. We do not know" (Freud 1924a: 160).

33 Freud develops these intuitions in the context of a comparison between Sophocles's *Oedipus Rex* and Shakespeare's *Hamlet* in *The Interpretation of Dreams* (Freud 1900: 264).

34 In "Civilized' Sexual Morality and Modern Nervous Illness," Freud argues that throughout human history one can distinguish three developmental phases of the sexual drive: a "polymorphous perverse" phase in which the sexual drive is free and not bound to the aim of reproduction; a second phase in which the sexual drive is repressed, with the exception of sexual activities that can serve reproduction; and a third phase in which only "legitimate" reproductive sexual activities are allowed (Freud 1908b: 189).

35 The final essay of *Totem and Taboo* and Freud's ideas on the acquisition of historical material can be situated in the context of the debate with Jung and his views on the relation between natural and cultural evolution relative to the development and differentiation of the libido (Vandermeersch 1991; Westerink 2009).

36 In another footnote from 1915 dealing with the incest barrier, we find a similar reasoning: "[t]he barrier against incest is probably among the historical acquisitions of humankind, and, like other moral taboos, has no doubt already become established in many persons by organic inheritance" (Freud 1905c: 225).

37 Freud refers to these insights in a footnote introduced in the 1920 edition (Ibid.: 226). On this issue, see also Fletcher (2013: 266–269).

38 Interestingly, in this case study he not only argues that the phylogenetically acquired material must await experiences before it can make itself felt but also adds that this acquired material can actually change the accidental experiences by filling the gaps and blind spots in these experiences; however, when this acquired material is not activated by actual experiences, it will spontaneously become productive through phantasies.

39 Although a closer analysis of the issue is beyond the scope of this book, we do want to mention the fact that in *Beyond the Pleasure Principle*, Freud almost exclusively refers to "death drives" (plural), whereas in *The Ego and the Id* and later texts he writes "death drive" (singular). In this chapter, we maintain this distinction.

3

BEYOND *THREE ESSAYS ON THE THEORY OF SEXUALITY*

Introduction

At the end of the previous chapter, we raised the question as to why Freud did not extensively introduce the Oedipus complex in the later editions of *Three Essays*. Why did Freud barely mention the Oedipus complex, which by then he considered to be the "shibboleth" of psychoanalytic theory? One could indeed legitimately claim that the third edition of *Three Essays* paves the way for the introduction of the famous complex, which was, as we already know, literally unthinkable in the editions from 1905 and 1910 given that infantile sexuality was still thought to be strictly autoerotic. As long as Freud considered infantile sexuality essentially non-objectal, oedipal constellations structurally belonged to puberty. This potentially changes when Freud introduces the notion of a diphasic object choice in 1915.

Yet Freud does not introduce the Oedipus complex in the third edition. Maybe this can be explained by the fact that at that time he was still of the opinion that "in childhood the combination of the component instincts and their subordination in the service of the genitals have been effected only very incompletely or not at all" (Freud 1905c: 199). The subordination of the component instincts in the service of the genitals seems indeed to be a necessary precondition for the Oedipus complex. This implies a (genital) libidinal investment in the parent of the opposite sex. In a footnote added in 1924, Freud refers to "The Infantile Genital Organisation." In this text, he explained that the two pre-genital organizations we previously discussed are followed by a third one "which already deserves to be described as genital." This means that it "presents a sexual object and some degree of sexual impulses upon that object" (Ibid.: 199–200, in note). This third libidinal phase, Freud continues, is differentiated from the final organization of sexual maturity in one essential respect: it knows only one kind of genitalia – the male. This is why Freud calls it "the phallic phase" (Ibid.; Freud 1923a: 142–145). It is only after the introduction of the phallic phase that Freud can introduce the Oedipus complex in the full sense of its meaning. The latter indeed implies that the little child can relate to a single person while its partial drives are already subsumed under the primacy of the genital organs.

All of this may explain why the Oedipus complex is mentioned for the first time in the 1920 version of *Three Essays*. But even then it remains a question as to why the "shibboleth" of psychoanalysis is discussed only in two footnotes (Freud 1905c: 226, in note). What explains this quasi-absence of the Oedipus complex in the later editions of *Three Essays*? This question is important because our efforts to understand it will confront us with crucial concepts that are lacking in Freud's theories of sexuality from 1905 and 1915. Without these crucial concepts – notably identification, ego ideal, conscience and superego formation, hatred, and guilt – the Oedipus complex cannot be properly articulated. It will turn out that some of these concepts cannot be properly understood until the introduction of the theory of the death drive(s) and life drives in *Beyond the Pleasure Principle* in 1919.[1] From this perspective, the fully established version of the Oedipus complex appears to be intrinsically linked to a new theory of the drives that never made its way into the last edition of *Three Essays*. In this chapter, we will thematize the problematic absence of the Oedipus complex in *Three Essays* and its relation to Freud's new theory of the drives. To do so, we first have to consider what the Oedipus complex is about and what it is supposed to achieve.

The father complex and the sadistic impulses

We cannot in the context of this book give a complete account of the (history of the) Oedipus complex in Freud's thinking, which deserves a detailed study in its own right. As we said earlier, references to Sophocles's Oedipus tragedy are present in Freud's work from the late 1890s. However, these references are only systematized into a psychological complex that structures the unconscious and that forms the basis of all psychopathology after the first publication of *Three Essays*. Even though there clearly are elements in Freud's study on Little Hans that anticipate the introduction of the Oedipus complex,[2] the publication that is particularly decisive for its introduction is the case study on the Rat Man. We already mentioned that Freud's clinical interest shifts after 1905 from hysteria to obsessional neurosis and psychosis. "Dora" was Freud's last case study of a hysterical patient. The study of the Rat Man illustrates Freud's renewed interest in the problematic of obsessional neurosis. It is only hereafter that Freud will start thematizing the Oedipus complex as the nuclear complex of all the psychoneuroses.

The introduction of the Oedipus complex and the systematic reflection on obsessional neuroses are two sides of the same coin. Indeed, the problems that play a crucial role in obsessional neurosis as Freud analyzes it after 1905 are intrinsically linked to the problems that structure the Oedipus complex. His obsessional patients confront Freud with the problems of antisocial and aggressive impulses, the sense of guilt, and the status of conscience (Freud 1907, 1909c) – issues that played only a minor role in his studies on hysteria. In the case of the Rat Man, Freud writes the following on this: "[w]hat is characteristic of this neurosis – what differentiates it from hysteria – is not, in my opinion, to be found in instinctual life but in the psychological field"; namely, the disintegration "into three personalities" (Ibid.: 248). Freud here articulates an intuition that he will soon further develop in his theory of narcissism and the study of melancholia: the significance of conscience (relative to the ego ideal, e.g., superego) as a psychic function that should be distinguished from the ego and the unconscious ("three personalities").

The problematics of aggression and the sense of guilt are central in the case of the Rat Man. According to Freud, his patient suffers from fits of rage and (unconscious) guilt feelings toward his father. To shed light on these symptomatic elements, Freud introduces the so-called father complex (Ibid.: 218). He claims that the successive rages of the Rat Man – against an old professor who occupies a room next to a nurse he fancies, against his fiancée, who stays with her grandmother instead of coming to him, etc. – are nothing but replays of an infantile scene of rage against his father, who had forbidden him to bite the maid. By interfering in the Rat Man's realization of his sexual (sadistic) activities, the father is the first object of a fit of rage, and Freud thinks that the old professor, the fiancée, and also some army officers are all basically substitutes for his father. The later accidental rages of the Rat Man are, according to Freud, essentially always directed toward the same object: his father. In Freud's view, these rages can therefore be interpreted in terms of a continuous hatred toward the father. This far from self-evident but important step is crucial (Haute & Geyskens 2016; Westerink 2016) because it determines the interpretation of the case and the role of the father: "[w]e may regard the repression of his infantile hatred of his father as the event which brought his whole subsequent career under the dominion of the neurosis" (Freud 1909c: 238). In other words, conflicting feelings[3] of love and hate toward the father are at the heart of the obsessional neurosis. The term *father complex* indicates this conflicting relation to the father, who is simultaneously loved and (unconsciously) hated because he had frustrated the Rat Man's sadistic impulses. The Rat Man's unconscious guilty feelings are basically seen as reaction formations against the persisting aggressive impulses toward the father. As regards the origin of and relation between love and hatred, Freud remarks that we know too little about these problematics to be able to draw conclusions. However, he does suggest that hatred can be seen as an unconscious form of a persisting sadistic impulse; that is, hatred is an expression of the sadistic component of the libido (Freud 1909c: 239–241).[4]

From its introduction in 1910 until the publication of *The Ego and the Id*, the Oedipus complex is more or less identical to the father complex or to what Freud later will call the "positive Oedipus complex." In this period – notably in *Totem and Taboo* – Freud systematically identifies the Oedipus complex with the rivalry between father and son over the possession of the mother.[5] In *Totem and Taboo*, this rivalry is predominantly described in terms of ambivalent feelings of hatred and love – a rivalry that culminates in parricide and the cannibalistic act of "identification."[6] The outcome of this drama is the "displacement" of ambivalent feelings onto a "substitute" for the father (the totem animal) (Freud 1912–1913: 128, 142), on the basis of which the prohibition of the mother as a sexual object can be internalized. In *Totem and Taboo*, for example, Freud writes on Little Hans:

> [h]e regarded his father (as he made all too clear) as a competitor for the favours of his mother, towards whom the obscure foreshadowings of his budding sexual wishes were aimed. Thus he was situated in the typical attitude of a male child towards his parents to which we have given the name of the "Oedipus complex" and which we regard in general as the nuclear complex of the neuroses.
>
> *(Freud 1912–1913: 129)*

We know already that at this point Freud did not yet consider these "budding sexual wishes" and this "typical attitude" in genital terms. But apart from this point, the father complex can easily be formulated in relation to the theory of the drives Freud was developing in the same period. The little child (boy) takes his mother as a sexual object and experiences his father as an obstacle to the realization of his sexual wishes, which explains the aggression against the father. Hence, this hatred can be understood from the perspective of the sadistic component inhabiting the drive from the outset – an idea Freud introduced in the third edition of his text. Important questions, however, remain. Can all hatred be fully understood from the sadistic component of the libido? And what exactly is "identification"? What are its psychodynamic implications, and what is its place in the Oedipus complex?

The Oedipus complex, identification, and ego ideal

In *The Ego and the Id*, published in 1923, we find what is generally considered the definitive version of the Oedipus complex. The complete Oedipus complex consists of a positive and a negative form:

> [c]loser study usually discloses the more complete Oedipus complex, which is twofold, positive and negative, and is due to the bisexuality originally present in children: that is to say, a boy has not merely an ambivalent attitude towards his father and an affectionate object-choice towards his mother, but at the same time he also behaves like a girl and displays an affectionate feminine attitude to his father and a corresponding jealousy and hostility towards his mother.
>
> *(Freud 1923b: 33)*

Interestingly enough, Freud considers this twofold structure of the Oedipus complex an expression of the constitutional bisexuality that, as we know, played a crucial role in the first editions of *Three Essays*. This means that Freud does not simply give up the theory of bisexuality in his later work, but rather that he subsumes it under his new oedipal theory of the neuroses. This is important to recognize, though not of crucial importance for the problems we want to solve in this chapter.

Of greater importance is the following: Freud writes in *The Ego and the Id* that we should in principle consider the presence of the complete Oedipus complex in all of us, and most certainly in neurotic patients. He further writes that with the dissolution of the complex

> the four trends of which it consists will group themselves in such a way as to produce a father-identification and a mother-identification. The father-identification will preserve the object-relation to the mother which belonged to the positive complex and will at the same time replace the object-relation to the father which belonged to the inverted complex: and the same will be true, *mutatis mutandis*, of the mother-identification.
>
> *(Ibid.: 34)*

It follows from this, Freud continues, that the most general outcome of the Oedipus complex is the formation of a "precipitate in the ego" that consists of these two identifications in some way united with each other. Freud identifies this "precipitate" with the superego that he had previously named the ego ideal.

Already in "On Narcissism" Freud postulated the necessity of this ego ideal that inherits infantile narcissism and without which the repression proceeding from the "self-respect of the ego" would be inconceivable. The ego ideal is not only a displacement of the subject's narcissism onto an ideal ego through which the narcissistic ideal of "perfection" can be maintained but notably also "an ideal in himself by which he measures his own ego" (Freud 1914a: 93). Freud continues by arguing that "a special psychical agency" – conscience – performs this task of measuring (Ibid.: 95–96). Indeed, Freud writes that there is a critical instance that protects the narcissistic satisfaction we can get from the ego ideal by repressing all psychic contents that contradict it. This critical instance, Freud writes in his text on narcissism, is the

> embodiment, first of parental criticism, and subsequently of that of society – a process which is repeated in what takes place when a tendency towards repression develops out of a prohibition or obstacle that came in the first instance from without.
>
> *(Ibid.: 96)*

But Freud does not explain in this seminal text how this division of the ego into two "personalities" comes about. He will further develop his views on this issue in his study on melancholia that was published in 1917.[7] In this text, Freud argues that a lost love object can be set up again inside the ego through narcissistic identification (Freud 1917: 249). This identification can be understood from the main constitutional factors that play a role in the etiology of melancholia: the narcissistic object choice and the ambivalence of feelings of love and hatred toward objects. According to Freud, the object choice is narcissistic when the object is chosen in the first place after the model of one's own self. The object is loved because it represents what the subject is, was, or would like to be. The object is hence not chosen for its capacity to satisfy the self-preservative needs of nutrition, care, and protection (anaclitic object choice), but rather for its capacity to represent the ego ideal and continue narcissistic self-love (Freud 1914a: 88–90). This narcissistic object choice helps us understand the withdrawal of libido into the ego that results from the shattered object relationship through actual loss (death) of, neglect by, or severe disappointment in the love object. The free libido is not displaced onto a substitute object but will be employed "to establish an identification of the ego with the abandoned object" (Freud 1917: 249). In other words, melancholia is first of all characterized by a specific reaction to the loss of (or disappointment in) an object; namely, an identification on the basis of a narcissistic object choice. Why does this process produce the severe and destructive self-reproaches that characterize melancholia? According to Freud, the identification with the lost object is not only a manner in which the love relationship need not be given up but also "an excellent opportunity for the ambivalence in love-relationships to make itself effective and come into the open" (Ibid.: 250–251). With the transformation of object loss into ego loss, the ambivalent feelings of love and hatred toward the object (which are "excessive" or "reinforced" in the case of melancholic patients) are also transformed and will manifest themselves in the split between the critical activity of the ego (conscience) and the ego as altered by identification. In this way, the destructive debasing of the ego and the self-tormenting through conscience that we find in melancholia can both be understood as forms of revenge on the original object. Through identification the individual turns against his or her own ego as if it were the lost love object.

> Thus the shadow of the object fell upon the ego, and the latter could henceforth be judged by a special agency, as though it were an object, the forsaken object. In this way, an object-loss was transformed into an ego-loss.
>
> *(Ibid.: 249)*

Melancholia therefore makes it possible to understand how one part of the ego turns against the other as a critical tribunal that we call conscience. Freud repeats these insights in the chapter on identification in his book *Group Psychology and the Analysis of the Ego* and also in *The Ego and the Id*. In both texts he identifies the critical function of conscience and the ego ideal. He writes:

> [o]n previous occasions ["On Narcissism," "Mourning and Melancholia"] we have been driven to the hypothesis that some such agency develops in our ego which may cut itself off from the rest of the ego and come into conflict with it. We have called it the "ego-ideal," and by way of functions we have ascribed to it self-observation, the moral conscience, the censorship of dreams, and the chief influence in repression.
>
> *(Freud 1921: 109–110)*

Additionally, in *The Ego and the Id*, Freud clearly states that the superego's later domination of the ego takes "the form of conscience or perhaps of an unconscious sense of guilt" (Freud 1923b: 35). This formation of the superego, and hence of conscience, is the most general outcome of the Oedipus complex.[8] Freud further reflects on its origin in *Group Psychology and the Analysis of the Ego* and *The Ego and the Id* by elaborating on the identification with what he usually calls the father of personal prehistory – though one could also call it "the parents" given that this identification precedes "definite knowledge of the difference between the sexes" (Ibid.: 31, in note).

According to Freud, this first identification is the most significant one in every individual. It is a derivative of the oral phase of the libido, and as such it is intrinsically ambivalent, for in this phase of the libido the object is assimilated by eating, and it is in this way annihilated. When in a later phase the (male) child develops a sexual object relation to his mother and he inevitably sees the father as a rival, the identification takes on a hostile allure and becomes identical to the wish to replace the father in his relation to the mother. In this way, this identification helps prepare the Oedipus complex (Freud 1921: 105, 1923b: 32). Freud writes both in *Group Psychology and the Analysis of the Ego* and *The Ego and the Id* that the primordial identification with the father precedes every object relation. But he also adds that the object choices with the father and the mother that characterize the first sexual period normally find their outcome in identifications that strengthen the primordial one: the relation to the object is replaced by an identification, as is the case in melancholia.

It is clear from our presentation so far that Freud's theory of identification and ego ideal, superego, and conscience formation runs parallel to the development of the Oedipus complex. The outcome of the latter, as thematized in *Group Psychology and the Analysis of the Ego* and *The Ego and the Id*, is simply inconceivable without a detailed theory of identification. It follows from this that inserting the Oedipus complex into the later editions of *Three Essays* would have implied treating the status and role of identification. The question we have to answer, then, is whether this would have been possible within the context of the model Freud used in the first editions of *Three Essays*.

Identification and sexuality

We know that in *Three Essays* Freud defends a strict distinction between (infantile) sexuality and self-preservation. But how can we situate identification in this dichotomy? Freud stresses in the first place that identification with love objects goes along with a desexualization, as in the case of the identification with the parents that is the outcome of the Oedipus complex. Identification, in other words, is a form of sublimation (Freud 1923b: 30). The relation between identification and sexuality is thus unclear from the outset. But the relation with sexuality is also problematic with regard to other types of identification that Freud distinguishes. In this context, he mentions the so-called psychic infection that occurs in boarding schools when, for example, one of the girls reacts with a hysterical fit to a letter she received from somebody she is secretly in love with. Such a letter might arouse jealousy in the other girls, who, as a consequence, "catch" the fit by psychic imitation. Freud writes:

> [t]he mechanism is that of identification based upon the possibility or desire of putting oneself in the same situation. The other girls would like to have a secret love affair too, and under the influence of a sense of guilt they also accept the suffering involved in it.
>
> (Freud 1921: 107)

What is interesting for us here is the fact that this identification takes place *with a person who is not an object of the sexual drive*. According to Freud, this is proven by the fact that this kind of imitation takes place even in circumstances where there is less pre-existing sympathy than between friends in a girls' school. "It would be wrong," Freud concludes, "to suppose that they take on the symptom out of sympathy. On the contrary, the sympathy only arises out of the identification" (Ibid.).[9] But does this mean that identification is not sexual in itself?

The problem we are addressing here is even clearer with regard to the identification with the father of the individual prehistory. Freud calls this identification "a typical identification" that prepares the Oedipus complex (Ibid.: 105). He writes that the young boy already takes his father as a model or an ideal in the pre-oedipal time. This identification plays a role in the prehistory of the Oedipus complex that it helps prepare. When the little boy notices that his father stands between him and his mother, the identification acquires a hostile character. Seen from this perspective, the identification indeed perfectly fits the Oedipus complex. Since this complex is supposed to be ambivalent from the outset, it can express both tenderness and a wish of elimination. Freud explains this ambivalence, as we know already, by calling this identification with the father a derivative of the oral phase of the libido in which the loved object is incorporated by eating it. But eating the object also implies a destruction of the object. The cannibal is, according to Freud, a good example of this: he loves his enemies so much that he eats them and does not eat those that he does not love (Ibid.: 105). This reference to the oral phase of the libido seems to justify the idea that the identification is in line with the sexual drive. But once again, things are more complicated than they first seem, for Freud at the same time distinguishes this identification from a choice for the father as an object. In *Group Psychology and the Analysis of the Ego*, he states the following on this topic:

> [i]dentification is known to psycho-analysis as the earliest expression of an emotional tie with another person. It plays a part in the early history of the Oedipus complex. A little boy will exhibit a special interest in his father; he would like to grow like him and be like him, and take his place everywhere. [. . .] At the same time as this identification with his father, or a little later, the boy has begun to develop a true object-cathexis towards his mother according

> to the attachment type. He then exhibits, therefore, two psychologically distinct ties: a straightforward sexual object-cathexis towards his mother and an identification with his father which takes him as his model. [. . .]
>
> In the first case one's father is what one would like to be and in the second he is what one would like to have. The distinction, that is, depends upon whether the tie attaches to the subject or to the object of the ego. *The former kind of tie is therefore already possible before any sexual object-choice has been made.*
>
> *(Ibid.: 105–106, emphasis ours)*

Since the sexual drive in the later versions of *Three Essays* is thought to be essentially object-related, these statements seem to imply that the "earliest expression of an emotional tie," which the identification is said to be, cannot be called "sexual" in any straightforward way. The little boy wants *to be like* the father, rather than *having* him as a sexual object. This implies that this "emotional tie," through identification, can already take place prior to any object relation. But if this is the case, the identification cannot be considered "sexual" given that Freud believes at this stage of his work that sexuality is structurally linked to an object. As a result, the relation can only be thought exclusively mimetic:[10] "[o]ne can only see that identification endeavors to mould a person's own ego after the fashion of the one that has been taken as a model" (Ibid.: 106). The problem now is this: the "mimetic" relation cannot properly be situated within the binary opposition between object-related sexuality and self-preservation as Freud originally articulated it in *Three Essays*. It is neither one nor the other (Borch-Jacobsen 1982). As a result, Freud's theory of identification transcends the dichotomy between sexual drives and the drives for self-preservation that determines the structure of *Three Essays*. Here we find the first important reason as to why Freud could not introduce the Oedipus complex in *Three Essays* without articulating a new theory of the drives in which the problem and status of identification at the basis of this complex could be properly situated.

Sexuality, aggression, and guilt

The character of Freud's original theory of the drives, as first articulated in 1905 and then later replaced by a more substantial theory in 1915, is insufficient for understanding different aspects of the Oedipus complex, and this insufficiency becomes even more obvious when we take the characteristics and functions of the superego (ego ideal, conscience) into account. We have already described that the formation of the superego implies that one part of the ego aggressively turns against the other. This aggression does not have an explosive character, as one sees, for example, in a fit of rage, but instead has a permanent character, as one sees in the case of hatred. This is in congruence with Freud's idea of the drive as a constant force that he introduces in "Instincts and Their Vicissitudes" (Freud 1915c: 118).[11]

According to Freud, the obsessional neurotic's unconscious feelings of guilt and the melancholic's self-reproaches find their origin in the strong tension between the ego and the ego ideal, i.e., superego. They are the expression of the condemnation of the ego by its critical faculty, conscience. In the case of obsessional neurosis and melancholia, "the ego ideal displays particular severity and often rages against the ego in a cruel fashion (Freud 1923b: 51). These pathologies show us in a magnified and exaggerated form that feelings of guilt are the effect of continuous aggressive impulses turned toward the ego; this characterizes the very nature of the superego. In obsessional neurosis, the patient cannot understand the origin of their unconscious feelings of guilt. Analysis then shows that the superego is under the spell of repressed processes of which the ego was not aware. These repressed processes justify the feelings of guilt: "the super-ego knew more than the ego about the unconscious id" (Ibid.: 51). More concretely, the ego was not aware of its aggressive impulses and phantasies toward the love object for which it is judged guilty by the superego.

In melancholia, however, the patient accepts both their guilt and the punishments they are subjected to. Freud writes:

> [i]n obsessional neurosis, what were in question were objectionable impulses which remained outside the ego, while in melancholia the object to which the super-ego's wrath applies has been taken into the ego through identification.
> *(Ibid.)*

With regard to melancholia, he says the following: "we find that the excessively strong superego which has obtained a hold upon consciousness rages against the ego with merciless violence" (Ibid.: 53). In this case, the superego regularly manages to push the ego to suicide (Ibid.). In obsessional neurosis, however, things are less clear and in a sense less extreme – suicide is seldom seen among obsessional neurotic patients. In fact, the obsessional neurotic person is well protected against the tendency toward self-destruction because "the object has been retained." What we witness here is a regression to the pre-genital, anal-sadistic organization, which explains the transformation of love impulses into impulses of aggression against an object that was always already invested with ambivalent feelings; this is what Freud had already shown in the case of the Rat Man. Freud writes that in obsessional neurosis these impulses remain in the Id. The ego does not adopt them. Precisely because they are ego-dystonic, the ego struggles against them by creating reaction formations and taking precautionary measures. Extreme tenderness, for instance, can hide excessive aggressive phantasies the ego is not conscious of. The superego, however, treats the ego as if it were responsible for them and acts accordingly. It chastises the destructive impulses and the ego that is supposed to be their agent (Ibid.). In both cases – melancholia and obsessional neurosis – the superego turns against the ego, which becomes the object of its aggression (hate). This aggression is at the basis of the unconscious feelings of guilt and self-reproaches that in these two pathologies dominate the clinical picture.

We know now the origin of the aggression directed toward the ego in melancholia and obsessional neurosis. However, we do not yet understand how the superego can express itself in such a ruthless and cruel way, which in melancholia often leads to suicide:

> so immense is the ego's self-love, which we have come to recognize as the primal state from which instinctual life proceeds, and so vast is the amount of narcissistic libido which we see liberated in the fear that emerges as a threat to life, that we cannot conceive how that ego can content to its own destruction.
>
> *(Freud 1917: 252)*

In the next sections, we will show that this problem inevitably leads to questions that cannot be answered within the framework of the libido theory that Freud defends in the 1905 and 1915 editions of *Three Essays*. To substantiate this claim, we will first turn our attention to Freud's explanation of the suicidal tendencies that make melancholia such an enigmatic and dangerous pathology.

Self-destructive hatred in obsessional neurosis and melancholia

The problem of how self-destruction and suicide are possible seems unsolvable within the context of the theory of the drives found in the first edition of *Three Essays*. If the drives seek only and exclusively satisfaction of needs (with the aim of self-preservation) or pleasurable sensations and excitations (sexuality) and avoid unpleasure, how, then, can we understand the extreme tendencies toward self-destruction that regularly characterize melancholia? Since aggression and hatred are hardly mentioned or thematized in the 1905 edition, it comes up short against the questions that need to be answered with regard to this problem, which shows itself in a magnified way in obsessional neurosis and melancholia but in fact concerns human nature more broadly. Freud amended his theory of sexuality in his 1915 "Instincts and Their Vicissitudes." In this text, he continues to stick to the opposition between sexual drives and drives for self-preservation, but he profoundly reformulates the nature of the sexual drives. With regard to these drives he now writes that they "go beyond the individual and have as their content the production of new individuals – that is, the preservation of the species" (Freud 1915: 125). In this way, Freud breaks away from the non-functional theory of sexuality that we found in the 1905 edition of the text. Sexuality becomes a reproductive function once again, a shift we discussed at length in the previous chapters. But in "Instincts and Their Vicissitudes," Freud tries to integrate the aggressive aspects of sexuality much more than before. We have already mentioned one important aspect of this integration. Freud in 1915 identifies the drive for mastery with the sadistic component of the sexual drive, and he writes that this sadistic component can also be turned against oneself (Ibid.: 127ff).

Freud further develops in this text a new theory on the origin of hatred and, more particularly, on the questions of how, under what circumstances, and with what implications love can turn into hatred and vice versa (Ibid.: 133). This question leads Freud to formulate the following hypothesis:

> the object is brought to the ego from the external world in the first instance by the instincts of self-preservation; and it cannot be denied that hating, too, originally characterized the relation of the ego to the alien external world with the stimuli it introduces.
>
> *(Ibid.: 136)*

Hence, "it seems, the external world, objects, and what is hated are identical" (Ibid.). According to Freud, any object brought to the "narcissistic ego" from the outside world pours out stimuli (*Reize*) that the person conceives as unpleasurable. Objects are primarily seen as hostile and anxiety-producing intrusions, and primal hatred therefore finds its first expressions in attempts to increase the distance between object and ego (e.g., through flight or destruction) – an idea that can be seen as the radical dismissal of the Darwinian notion of a primary social instinct for "sympathy" or attachment. However, if such an alien, hated object turns out to be a source of pleasure, it will become loved and also "incorporated into the ego." If this pleasure for some reason (such as a conflict) then turns into unpleasure, the loved object will be distanced from the ego and will once again become the object of hatred (Ibid.: 137).

In "Mourning and Melancholia," Freud refers to this new theory to understand the enigmatic suicidal tendencies and self-destruction that characterize melancholia. In the first moment, Freud writes that the loss of the loved object is a privileged moment for the ambivalence of the love relations to become manifest. The melancholic patient tries to save his or her relation with the object by identifying with it. This narcissistic identification at the basis of melancholia explains why the hatred that had been directed toward the lost object now turns toward the ego:

> [t]he self-tormenting in melancholia, which is without doubt enjoyable, signifies, just like the corresponding phenomenon in obsessional neurosis, a satisfaction of trends of sadism and hate which relate to an object, and which have been turned round upon the subject's own self in the ways we have been discussing.
>
> *(Freud 1917: 251)*

This means not only that melancholia is characterized by an identification with the lost object but also that this identification is accompanied by a regression to the anal-sadistic phase under the influence of the ambivalence conflict: "[i]t is this sadism alone that solves the riddle of the tendency to suicide which makes melancholia so interesting" (Freud 1917: 252). Freud seems to be talking here about sadism as an intrinsic component of sexuality. However, recall that for Freud, identification is accompanied by a desexualization or sublimation of the drive. Hence, the suicidal tendencies under consideration find their origin in sublimated sadistic tendencies that search for satisfaction. This would imply that the suicidal tendencies in melancholia can be explained from the perspective of the vicissitudes of the sexual drive alone.

But this is not Freud's last word on the matter. Indeed, in the following paragraph, Freud links these sadistic (sexual) tendencies to the theory of the origin of hatred we mentioned just a moment ago:

> [t]he analysis of melancholia now shows that the ego can kill itself only if, owing to the return of the object-cathexis, it can treat itself as an object – if it is able to direct against itself the hostility which relates to an object *and which represents the ego's original reaction to objects in the external world.*
>
> *(Ibid., emphasis ours)*

Freud does not really explain in "Mourning and Melancholia" how the relation between the regression to the sadistic phase and the primal hatred toward the object can be conceived. But in "Instincts and Their Vicissitudes," to which Freud here refers, he states that the regression strengthens the primal hatred toward the object and hence toward the ego that identifies with it (Freud 1915: 139). What Freud seems to imply here is that the merging of sadistic (libidinal) impulses and hatred will allow us to understand and explain the self-destructive tendencies typical of the melancholic pathology.

Could we not then conclude from all this that Freud's 1915 theory of the drives is a sufficient framework for understanding the self-destructive tendencies that characterize melancholia and that can drive the ego to suicide? It is true that Freud did not integrate all the aspects of this theory into the third edition of *Three Essays*, but the aspects that he did not mention do not contradict the overall picture of *Three Essays*. Or, in other words, even though Freud did not mention his new theory of hatred in the 1915 *Three Essays*, it is entirely compatible with the overall line of reasoning in the text given that its starting point is the strict opposition between sexual drives and drives for self-preservation. This opposition is at the basis of the logic that governs *Three Essays*. Then why did we claim that Freud's original theory of the drives was incapable of doing justice to the characteristics and functions of the superego that is the main outcome of the Oedipus complex?

The problem of identification and a new theory of the drives

We explained how the theory of the origin of hatred that Freud develops in "Instincts and their Vicissitudes" allows for an explanation of the aggressive tendencies of the superego against the ego. Melancholia and obsessional neurosis exemplify this in a magnified way. However, what still remains unexplained in this theory is the very origin of the superego. Freud claims that the superego finds its origin in the identification with the prehistoric father (parents) and that it is further strengthened by the replacement of the early object choices for the father and the mother with a narcissistic identification, for which melancholia gives us a model. But this model or paradigm seems to contradict the basic assumptions of Freud's early theory of the sexual drives. The problem Freud faces here is the following: if the sexual drive only looks for pleasure, as he keeps insisting, and if the object furthermore is the most variable aspect of the drive (Freud 1915: 122–123), then how can we understand that the drive apparently has a hard time giving up the objects in which it has invested? Indeed, in contradistinction to what we would expect on the basis of Freud's early theories, both mourning and melancholia show us that the libido is quite reluctant to give up its love objects. In a short text called "On Transience," Freud writes in regard to this that "[w]e only see that libido clings to its objects and will not renounce those that are lost even when a substitute lies really to hand. Such then is mourning." He adds to this the following: "[m]ourning over the loss of something that we have loved or admired seems so natural to the layman that he regards it as self-evident. But to psychologists mourning is a great riddle" (Freud 1916: 306–307). We now see that the psychologist's perplexity is caused by a problematic theory of the drives.

In the first edition of *Three Essays*, Freud mentioned the "need for variation" as a basic characteristic of the sexual drive. Even if this qualification disappeared in the fourth edition of our text, it is in complete agreement with the overall picture Freud gives of the sexual drive in all the editions of *Three Essays*: the libido searches for pleasure (or avoids unpleasure), and the object is only a means to realize that goal. From the perspective of the libido – at least if we follow Freud – an object should be easily replaceable with another when the search for pleasure obliges a person to do so. In the 1905 edition, Freud mentions only one exception to this general rule: the libido can get fixated on an earlier source of pleasure. That is exactly what happens in the different perversions (Freud 1905a: 18, 90). But in this case, the motivation of the libido concerns pleasure and not the object that procures it (or not). What we learn from mourning and melancholia is in a certain sense the opposite: it is the object we cannot let go, rather than the pleasure a person once experienced in relation to it. How much easier would life be if one could simply replace a deceased partner, who can no longer be a source of pleasure, with another?[12]

The problem we are confronted with here concerns more than just the relation between a person and present objects in the outside world. In fact, the studies of narcissism and melancholia show that objects are identified with the ego such that they continue to be an inner source of unpleasure, notably through the inner representation of such objects; that is, through conscience. The "conflict" between the ego and the lost love object is here replaced by a continuous inner conflict between the ego and a critical agency producing self-reproach. In *The Ego and the Id*, Freud argues that it is probably only through identification that the drives are prepared to give up their objects (Freud 1923b: 29). But at what cost? Melancholia shows us in an exaggerated manner that the price paid is the most severe self-criticism, i.e., the wrath of the superego turning the sadistic and hateful impulses toward the ego. Identification and the formation of an inner critical agency imply the continuation of constant inner conflict and a sense of guilt, but how do we explain the fact that these identification processes come to overrule the pleasure principle? If identification can be defined in terms of the continuation of a relation with an object *at all costs*, the question becomes which (physiological or) psychic principles or dynamics can explain and justify the inherent discarding of the pleasure principle. This question confronts Freud with a riddle that he will only be able to "solve" after fundamentally reconsidering his drive theory.

The opposition between the sexual and self-preservation drives determines the structure of *Three Essays* from its first until its last edition. Freud never changes this aspect of his text, although the interpretation of the two drives does evolve over time. In his 1920 *Beyond the Pleasure Principle*, Freud replaces this opposition with a new one between the death and life drives.[13] As we mentioned in the introduction to this chapter, there are only a few references in footnotes to this text in the later editions of *Three Essays*. In this respect, these references resemble the references to the Oedipus complex, which also never received a structural place in our text.

The introduction of this new theory of the drives is of crucial importance because it allowed Freud to solve the problem we just articulated.[14] Indeed, in the fourth chapter on "Two Classes of Instincts" in *The Ego and the Id*, Freud writes the following:

> [t]he other case will be recollected, in which the ego deals with the first object-cathexes of the id (and certainly with later ones too) by taking over the libido from them into itself and binding it to the alteration of the ego produced by means of identification. The transformation [of erotic libido] into ego-libido of course involves an abandonment of sexual aims, a desexualization. In any case this throws light upon an important function of the ego in its relation to Eros. By thus getting hold of the libido from the object-cathexes, setting itself up as sole love-object, and desexualizing or sublimating the libido of the id, the ego is working in opposition of the purposes of Eros and placing itself at the service of the opposing instinctual forces.
>
> *(Freud 1923b: 45–46)*

We have already discussed the relation between narcissistic identification and desexualization. In the passage we just quoted, Freud adds that this desexualization or sublimation happens in the service of hostile impulses – or what in this context comes down to the same thing – of the death drive, as opposed to Eros. How can we understand this enigmatic statement that links narcissistic identification and the desexualization that accompanies it to the death drive?

Taking up the problematic of *Beyond the Pleasure Principle*, Freud distinguishes in *The Ego and the Id* between the life drives or Eros and the death drive. About Eros he writes: "we are supposed that Eros, by bringing about a more and more far-reaching combination of the particles into which living substance is dispersed, aims at complicating life and at the same time, of course, at preserving it" (Freud 1923b: 40). As such, Eros contains both the uninhibited sexual drives and the drive for self-preservation; that is to say, the two poles of the initial opposition that determines the argumentation in *Three Essays* (Ibid.).[15] One could say that Eros contains the two progressive tendencies that underlie every physiological and psychological development of a person. In this sense, the conceptualization of Eros contributes to Freud's turn toward a developmental perspective on the human being.

Eros stands over and against the death drives. Freud discovers these drives in the compulsion to repeat that characterizes human existence and that operates independently of the pleasure principle.[16] This compulsion to repeat is witnessed in dreams of patients suffering from war neurosis and dreams that repeatedly bring a person back into the situation of an accident (Freud 1920: 12–13). The compulsion to repeat is also found in a child's play, accidently witnessed one day by Freud, in which the child repeatedly stages the distressing and clearly unpleasurable experience of the mother's departure (Ibid.: 14–16). Freud finds another example in his neurotic patient's compulsion to repeat repressed material (that is, experiences that include no possibility of pleasure) as a contemporary unpleasurable experience instead of remembering it as an experience from the past (Ibid.: 18–20). We cannot go into all the details of this difficult notion of the compulsion to repeat, as found in these very different examples, and of the complex way in which this compulsion to repeat is related to the drives. We limit ourselves to some elementary aspects of it. Our main goal here is simply to understand the link between the process of identification and the new theory of the drives. The dreams of traumatized persons, the child's play, and the "negative therapeutic reaction" that refers to the stubborn refusal of some patients to change (i.e., to get "cured") are, in Freud's view, striking examples of the fact that human existence cannot be understood from the perspective of the pleasure principle alone. Indeed, these dreams, plays, and reactions do not and cannot bring any pleasure to the individuals concerned. They are not motivated by pleasure, and for that reason the conception of fixation that we find in *Three Essays* and that we have already discussed does not suffice to understand these phenomena. Quite the contrary, they testify to a principle of inertia and reduction of tension that inhabits the human being as such and that opposes the forces of Eros – the life drives that produce excitation (tension).[17] Repetition is presented as "a universal attribute of drives." More precisely, it is an instinctual aspect of all organic life: "an urge inherent in organic life to restore an earlier state of things" (Ibid.: 36).[18] While the life drives try to complicate life and in doing so inevitably strive for change and renewal, the death drives refuse any development. The "organic" compulsion to repeat expresses the internal refusal of any change: it is "the conservative nature of living substance" (Ibid.; Fletcher 2013: 303–307). This force is not external to the movement of life. It is not an external barrier that opposes itself from the outside to the force of Eros. It indicates, on the contrary, an aspect of human nature that, so to speak, is already dead, while one is still alive.

From here the link Freud establishes between (narcissistic) identification and the death drives becomes intelligible. The ego identifies with the love objects because it does not want to lose them, because it wants to continue the attachment ("strong fixation," "pertinacity") to these objects or – what amounts to the same – because it does not want to change by choosing a new object. In turning itself into a love object of the Id, the ego allows the Id to stick to its old loves – it is a *continuation* of attachment through *regression* to original narcissism, i.e., to narcissistic identification (Freud 1917: 249). And it is these aspects of melancholia that point toward "an overcoming of the instinct which compels every living thing to cling to life" (Ibid.: 246). Whereas Eros and the pleasure principle push the individual to new objects, further development, and greater complexity, the (narcissistic) identification we are discussing here is more in line with the principle of inertia that Freud associates with the death drive.

As we already know, this identification furthermore implies sublimation or desexualization.[19] This desexualization allows us to understand how the principle of inertia, of which the identification is an expression, leads toward the (auto-)aggression that characterizes the superego. The aggression that is part of the ambivalent relation toward the love object can no longer be contained or "bound" by Eros as before. Desexualization initiates a defusion of erotic and aggressive impulses that, according to Freud, explains the cruel and demanding aspects of conscience.[20] And it is in this sense that Freud can refer to melancholia in terms of "a pure culture of the death instinct" (Freud 1923b: 53); that is, sadism and hatred become self-destructive in a fatal way on the basis of an identification with an object that cannot be given up.[21]

In his 1924 text on masochism, Freud will further explore the fusion and defusion of erotic and aggressive impulses. Freud argues that his theory of the death drives sheds new light on the origins of masochism. Whereas a large part of the death drive will be deferred to external objects (primal hatred, drive for mastery) or put directly into the service of the sexual function (sadism), another part will "remain in the organism," and "with the help of the accompanying sexual excitation described above, becomes libidinally bound there" (Freud 1924a: 163–164). This results in what Freud calls erogenous masochism. It is starting from this notion that he will also conceptualize moral masochism; that is, a form of masochism characterized by severe self-punishment that makes use of the superego that was established through identification. According to Freud, this moral masochism should not be understood as originating from an object relation, but rather as a continuation of the death drive that remains in the organism and expresses itself as a need for punishment and pain. In a footnote in the 1924 edition of *Three Essays*, Freud refers to these new ideas on masochism but without explicitly mentioning the theory of the death drive that led him to these new insights (Freud 1905c: 158).

Conclusion

We wondered, in this final chapter of our book on *Three Essays*, why some of Freud's most decisive findings are absent from the text. The main theme that is virtually lacking in *Three Essays* is the Oedipus complex. This has come as a surprise.[22] Does Freud himself not call it the "shibboleth" of psychoanalysis, and do most post-Freudian theorists not reread the whole development of Freudian thinking as a progressive discovery of this complex? Why, then, is the Oedipus complex hardly mentioned in Freud's most programmatic text on the theory of sexuality? And what can we learn from this absence?

Freud writes that the formation of the superego is the most general outcome of the Oedipus complex. This formation cannot be understood apart from a theory of identification. Indeed, it is melancholic identification as grounded in narcissistic object choice that, according to Freud, exemplifies the psychic process at the basis of the creation of the superego. Freud develops his theory of identification in *Group Psychology and the Analysis of the Ego* and *The Ego and the Id*, both of which appeared just prior to the publication of the last edition of *Three Essays*. We have shown how and why it is hard to reconcile this theory of identification with Freud's early theory, whose starting point is the strict opposition between the sexual drives and the drive for self-preservation as the basic motivational forces of human existence. Indeed, it turns out that identification cannot be reduced to either sexuality or self-preservation. The problematic relation between Freud's theory of identification and the early theory of the drives becomes particularly clear with regard to melancholic identification. Indeed, in melancholy the individual identifies with a lost object because it does not want to give it up. But how can we explain this tendency if the sexual drive seeks only pleasure and if the object is its most variable aspect? Clearly, Freud's early theory of the (sexual) drives is unable to explain these problems. This changes only when Freud introduces a new theory of the drives in *Beyond the Pleasure Principle* and *The Ego and the Id*. From then on, he replaces the opposition between sexual drives and the drive for self-preservation with an opposition between the life and death drives. Freud now interprets the conservative character of melancholic identification and the aggressiveness characterizing the superego as expressions of the death drive and the defusion of the aggressive and erotic drives, respectively.

The Oedipus complex brings the hysterical model that governs *Three Essays* to its ultimate limits. It requires a "paradigmatic shift" that Freud established in the early 1920s, notably in *The Ego and the Id*. This new paradigm contradicted the old in such a fundamental way that Freud could no longer integrate it into *Three Essays* without writing a completely new text.

Notes

1 Although a closer analysis of the issue is beyond the scope of this book, we do want to mention the fact that in *Beyond the Pleasure Principle,* Freud almost exclusively refers to "death drives" (plural) whereas in *The Ego and the Id* and later texts he writes "death drive" (singular). In this chapter, we maintain this distinction.

2 In the case study of Little Hans, Freud refers to the boy as "a little Oedipus" (Freud 1909a: 111); that is, as a boy who wants his father "out of the way" so that he can be alone with his mother and enjoy her cutaneous contact. Freud refers here to the Oedipus myth merely for its emblematic value. There is no mention here of the term "identification" (with the father).

3 In the Rat Man case study, Freud does not use the term *ambivalence* to describe the conflicting feelings of love and hatred. The concept of ambivalence was only first introduced in 1911 by Eugen Bleuler in the context of his studies on schizophrenia. Freud

adopts this concept in 1912 (Freud 1912: 106, 1912–1913: 29ff). In the 1915 edition of *Three Essays*, Freud uses the term to describe the currents of activity and passivity (Freud 1905c: 199). Notably, in the study on melancholia, Freud points out the significance of constitutional and accidental ambivalent feelings of love and hatred in human psychic life (Freud 1917: 256–258).

4 In the 1905 *Three Essays*, Freud had already suggested this without further explanation: "[i]t is also through this connection between libido and cruelty that the transformation of love into hate takes place, as does the transformation of affectionate into hostile stirrings, which is characteristic of a great number of cases of neurosis" (Freud 1905a: 27).

5 The case of the Wolf Man is often referred to as the case par excellence in which Freud provides clinical evidence of the Oedipus complex. It is a remarkable fact, however, that in this case study the Oedipus complex as such is only mentioned a few times, notably in the final section of the text, where Freud discusses the issue of inherited phylogenetic material (Freud 1918: 119). See also the previous chapter.

6 We note here that in *Totem and Taboo* Freud only mentions the term *identification* in the context of the son's act of devouring the father.

7 In the period in which Freud wrote his study on melancholia, the status of the concept of melancholia in the contemporary psychiatric literature was contested. Most importantly, Kraepelin, in the various editions of his textbook, had progressively started replacing the concept of melancholia with depression. And whereas he had initially seen melancholia as an important nosological category, he nuances this view in later editions. Moreover, Kraepelin had listed melancholia under the heading of endogenetic pathologies, thus sharply distinguishing melancholia from psychogenetic pathologies. Freud is clearly aware of this contestation when writing that the "definition fluctuates even in descriptive psychiatry" (Freud 1917: 243). Nevertheless, he chooses to maintain the concept and aims to extend psychoanalysis to the study of melancholia as well (as he had done a few years earlier in the case of paraphrenia [Schreber]) by exploring the psychogenetic aspects of a group of cases.

8 Freud sometimes distinguishes the superego from the ego ideal that represents the ideals to which the ego must correspond. In the texts we are analyzing here, the ego ideal is just an aspect of the superego that is further identified with the critical instance that scrutinizes the ego: conscience.

9 Again, we notice here that Freud does not explain sympathy from a social drive, as Darwin did.

10 See, on this topic, M. Borch-Jacobsen, *The Freudian Subject*, Stanford University Press, Stanford, 1988.

11 In the 1905 *Three Essays*, we do not yet find the idea that the drive is a "constant force." It is only first in "Instincts and Their Vicissitudes" that Freud makes a fundamental distinction between stimulus (*Reiz*) and drive: "all that is essential in a stimulus is covered if we assume that it operates with a single impact, so that it can be is posed of by a single expedient action. [. . .] An instinct, on the other hand, never operates as a force giving a *momentary* impact but always as a *constant* one" (Freud 1915: 118).

12 The fact that the "need for variation" was deleted in the 1920 edition can probably be seen as a result of the problem mourning and melancholia confronted Freud with: the continuation of the relation with a lost object through identification.

13 In an article that analyzes the complex realization of *Beyond the Pleasure Principle* in 1919–1920, Ulrike May-Tolzmann shows that the theory of the life and death drives (chapter 6 of that text) was first introduced only in the final version of the text. In the original draft from 1919, these concepts were absent (May-Tolzmann 2015b).

14 From the perspective of later texts like *Civilization and Its Discontents*, one might be tempted to argue that the theory of the death drives was introduced to provide a general theory of aggression. Indeed, in this major text Freud refers to the "blindest fury of destructiveness" as a manifestation of a drive of destruction that is "the derivative and main representative of the death instinct" (Freud 1930: 121–122). This interpretation

of the death drives as drive for destruction, however, cannot be found in *Beyond the Pleasure Principle* as such – elaborations on rage and hatred are practically absent in that text. (Freud elaborated only on the sadistic component of the drive.) One could argue that the idea of a "blindest fury of destructiveness" results from a reconsideration of the primal hatred as depicted in "Instincts and Their Vicissitudes": the most "primitive" aggression is maybe not the hatred that reacts against an object that causes unpleasure but a rage (*Wut*) that seeks an object to release tension (Moyaert 2014; Westerink 2016).

15 We should notice here that Eros as the drive toward coalescence with objects is at odds with the 1905 depiction of infantile sexuality as autoerotic and without object. In other words, the concept of Eros fundamentally undermines the 1905 theory of infantile sexuality. However, it does support the conceptualization of adult sexuality.

16 As early as the 1905 edition of *Three Essays*, Freud is already puzzled by the question of the "unknown origin" of a compulsion to repeat, which he further articulates in terms of a "pertinacity or susceptibility to fixation" in both neuroses and perversions that fails to "prescribe the paths to be taken by the sexual drive," i.e., fixations and repetitions that do not produce pleasure (Freud 1905a: 89).

17 For a more detailed account, see Moyaert 2014 and Bernet 2013.

18 In melancholia, this "organic" aspect can be witnessed in sleeplessness and the refusal to take nourishment (Freud 1917: 246).

19 For the complex relation between sublimation and desexualization in the work of Freud, see Moyaert 1994 and De Block 2004.

20 On this, Freud writes: "[t]he super-ego arises, as we know, from an identification with the father taken as a model. Every such identification is in the nature of a desexualization or even of a sublimation. It now seems as though when a transformation of this kind takes place, an instinctual defusion occurs at the same time. After sublimation, the erotic component no longer has the power to bind the whole of the destructiveness that was combined with it, and this is released in the form of an inclination to aggression and destruction. This defusion would be the source of the general character of harshness and cruelty by the ideal – its dictatorial 'Thou shalt'" (Freud 1923b: 44–45).

21 We agree on this point with Laplanche that "the essential dimension of the affirmation of a death drive lies not in the discovery of aggressiveness" but "in the idea that the aggressiveness is first of all directed against the subject and, as it were, *stagnant within him*" (Laplanche 1976: 86, emphasis ours). This is contrary to Lear (and others), who interprets the death drive as a drive toward self-destruction that needs deflection toward external objects to avoid this self-destruction. Aggression is here a defense against self-destructive tendencies (Lear 2005: 160–162). What Lear has clearly overlooked is the significance of Freud's theory of melancholia for the conceptualization of the death drive (De Vleminck 2013).

22 So much so that some just explain its logic while constantly referring to the "absent" complex (Quinodoz 2005: 52–65).

THE ACTUALITY OF FREUD'S *THREE ESSAYS ON THE THEORY OF SEXUALITY*

In our introduction, we mentioned Freud's own appreciation of the relation between the different editions of *Three Essays*. In the preface to the second edition, he writes: "what was imperfect may be replaced by something better." Strictly speaking, this statement applies only to the relation between the first two editions, but Freud clearly has a tendency to generalize this interpretation to his whole work. This tendency becomes notably apparent in his writings concerning the history of psychoanalysis. In "On the History of the Psycho-analytic Movement," for example, he writes that on the way toward a proper theory, "a mistaken idea had to be overcome which might have been almost fatal to the young science." This "mistaken idea" refers to the so-called seduction theory and "hysterical subjects tracing their symptoms to traumas that are fictitious" (Freud 1914b: 17). And in "An Autobiographical Study," he denies that the stories of seduction his patients told him in the early years were his own "suggestions." This time, Freud adds the claim that it was in these stories that he first encountered the Oedipus complex but that, at the time, he was not yet familiar with its phantasmatic disguise (Freud 1925: 33–34). Freud thus suggests that his thinking followed a continuous and progressive development from beginning to end. "Psychoanalysis," writes Freud, "is my creation," adding:

> I consider myself justified in maintaining that even today no one can know better than I do what psychoanalysis is, how it differs from other ways of investigating the life of the mind, and precisely what should be called psychoanalysis and what would better be described by some other name.
>
> *(Freud 1914b: 7)*

This creation consists of a progressive movement, of "digging deeper"[1] and "removing disguises" – two metaphors that point toward something like a hidden "truth" that was always waiting to be found. This fuels the idea that whenever we are referring to "Freud," we are referring to a unified and refined subject at the origin of the *Standard Edition of the Works of Sigmund Freud* that progressively articulates what it always already wanted to say, albeit implicitly and without clearly realizing it from the outset.[2] This presentation is inevitably teleological: the "truth" of Freudian thinking lies in Freud's last works, for which the early works serve as preparation. In such a view there is, at least in principle, no room for contradictions that cannot be undone, let alone for the idea that an author does not really "found," "own," or "control" their *oeuvre*.

Our reading of the different editions of Freud's *Three Essays* contradicts the view of Freudian thought as a progressively developed, coherent unity controlled by its author. It consists of an analysis of the architecture, reasoning, and concepts present in these editions. Already in the first edition of *Three Essays* Freud defends different positions that are hard to reconcile. The first two parts of this first edition articulate the view that sexuality is exclusively about a search for autoerotic pleasure, for which the object is purely instrumental. But at the beginning of the third essay, Freud articulates sexuality in terms of reproductive function, as most of his contemporaries did. Davidson writes in this respect that in the third part of *Three Essays*, Freud is the victim of the "mentality" of his day, from which he could not completely escape (Davidson 2001: 91). Does this mean that the third part of *Three Essays* does not contain the "real" Freud? Even in the first two essays, there are tensions and obscurities that are difficult to resolve. How, for example, can we understand the voyeuristic drive if infantile sexuality is intrinsically autoerotic? And how can the idea that the caregiver takes the child as a "full-fledged sexual object" be reconciled with a purely physiological approach to sexuality? Moreover, the first edition says hardly anything about the status of aggressiveness in human sexuality. No wonder the treatment of sadomasochism was (and could not but be) insufficient in this edition.

Several of the major controversies in debates with his earliest followers stem from the problems, tensions, and obscurities in Freud's 1905 theory of infantile sexuality. One might be tempted to agree with Freud's account of these controversies, which states that Adler's and Jung's positions were basically "heresies," amounting to rejections of the psychoanalytic "doctrine" (Freud 1914b). The importance of these controversies, however, does not lie in the demarcation of doctrines and school formations. On a more fundamental level, these controversies are situated within the field Freud had opened up in *Three Essays*. The questions raised by Adler and Jung can be seen as inquiries into the unresolved tensions and obscurities in Freud's text. Adler's elaborations of sexual aggression (Adler 1908) were based on the unsatisfactory accounts of sadism and the drive for mastery in *Three Essays*. More importantly, it was Jung who identified a few fundamental problems unresolved by Freud (Jung 1912a, 1912b; Vandermeersch 1991). Can one identify the autoerotic pleasure discovered in breastfeeding and repeated in sensual sucking as "sexual" when the concept of sexuality is actually derived from an adult constellation in which the genital drive can be seen as distinct from tendencies toward self-preservation? Is not the identification of an infantile sexual drive a projection of a differentiated "libido" in adult life? What is the libido exactly? Can it be defined in purely physiological terms or is there also a "psychological" component in the form of a "will" or "passionate desire"? Why does Freud stubbornly cling to a drive dichotomy when he himself at the same time undermines this idea when speaking of "a – or one – drive (*ein 'Trieb'*) that *becomes* sexual" (see p. 20, emphasis ours) or suggesting that not all drives – the drive for mastery or the drive for knowledge, for instance – can be reduced to the two original tendencies of a desire for food and a sexual drive. Further, can the relation between ontogenesis and phylogenesis be adequately addressed in a model that solely focuses on the moral aspects of culture while at the same time describing the relation between individual and culture as a scene of conflict? It is questions such as these that are at the heart of the field of problems addressed by Freud in *Three Essays*.

In the later editions of *Three Essays*, Freud tried to solve these tensions and to overcome manifest contradictions by introducing a developmental perspective partly inherited from his pupils (Abraham and Jung) and by introducing the notion of the diphasic object choice. In so doing, he moved the overall perspective of the text in a more "conservative," i.e., heteronormative, direction. But because he did not at the same time drastically change the first version of the text, the contradictions and tensions remained and became even more apparent. How, for instance, can we reconcile the idea that infantile sexuality is autoerotic and can be described in purely physiological terms with the idea that it is objectal from the outset?

It is not just that the first edition of *Three Essays* contains tensions and obscurities or manifests contradictions and questions that needed to be resolved in the later editions. The reader is also surprised by the absence of some key notions from Freudian psychoanalysis. The main example of such an absence is no doubt the Oedipus complex, which is mentioned only twice in the last editions and only in two footnotes. In most secondary literature, this absence is interpreted in line with Freud's self-interpretation, which we have already mentioned: the reference to an Oedipus complex was already implicitly present in the 1905 edition and only needed to be rendered explicit later on; it was perhaps still buried under other layers but was nevertheless already there, and consequently there is no discontinuity. But does such an interpretation make sense? Indeed, the idea that infantile sexuality is autoerotic does not leave room for the famous complex. The latter presupposes at least the possibility of a (phantasmatic) relation to the parents of both sexes as objects of the sexual drive. It comes as no surprise, then, that there is no mention of the Oedipus complex at all in this first edition. It was literally unthinkable given that infantile sexuality was conceived in exclusively physiological and non-objectal terms. On top of this, Freud never removed the passages on autoerotism from the later editions.

It is thus abundantly clear that the different editions of *Three Essays* cannot be read as a progressive deployment of intuitions that were present from the outset in disguised form, buried, or imperfectly articulated. Quite the contrary, the text contains a series of contradictions that cannot be resolved within the paradigm at hand. It is even quite unclear *who speaks* in the different passages of the texts. Most evidently, it is not a unified subject with the name "Sigmund Freud," who tries to express what he "really intents to say." There is no "unified thought" that can be reconstructed through the interpretation of the text.[3] Freud's claim that "psychoanalysis is my creation" is merely an argument from authority. The "officially approved" final version of *Three Essays on the Theory of Sexuality* must instead be read as a collage, a palimpsest of texts from different periods of Freud's intellectual development. Quite often, one text overwrites another, so that the latter disappears from view and is "forgotten." Contradictions and tensions are introduced or strengthened in the process, so that *Three Essays* becomes a very enigmatic document. The final text cannot be understood on the model of archaeological excavation as a progressive uncovering of the always already potentially or latently hidden oedipal core. Rather, this version buries an original version under later layers of fragments.

If we leave the idea behind that the different editions of *Three Essays* contain the progressive unfurling of a consistent and coherent body of thought belonging to a unified subject, we can begin to see them in a more fruitful and productive way. Indeed, *Three Essays* articulates not so much a "grand theory" on human sexuality but a problematic field of related questions that can be studied as such. From this perspective, the main task of the reader is not to undo the contradictions, uncertainties, and tensions we have mentioned in this book. Instead, we have to map and articulate the different (contradictory) positions at hand, the problems to which they are related, and the contexts in which they occur. In this way, even the questions and tensions become food for thought insofar as they highlight the manifold fundamental and philosophically relevant problems Freud was facing in the different editions of his text. This allows Freudian psychoanalysis to become once again a source of inspiration for a *contemporary philosophical anthropology*, rather than a "doctrine" of definitive answers.

Instead of a doctrine and a coherent theory, we find in *Three Essays* ambiguities and tensions oscillating between the poles of a radical critique of a heteronormative functional approach to sexuality on the one hand and a defense of a "normal" heterosexual organization of adult sexuality on the other. These poles can also be identified in the reception of Freudian thought. Herbert Marcuse's 1955 *Eros and Civilization*, for instance, was an influential Freudo-Marxist critique of oppressive and sexually repressive capitalist power structures in contemporary Western societies (Marcuse 1955; Müller-Funk 2016). This text was an inspiration for movements in the 1960s and 1970s that strove for sexual liberation. However, in that same period, we can also witness the rise of a powerful critique of Freudian thought as an oedipal theory that basically legitimized fatherly authority, cultural guilt, and conscience formations, and of course the nuclear family, with its traditional division of roles. Deleuze and Guattari's *Anti-Oedipe* (Deleuze & Guattari 1972) and Foucault's critique of the juridical character of the oedipal law (Foucault 1978, 1985) are likely among the most important of the philosophical critiques of psychoanalytic theory. The idea that psychoanalysis defends an intrinsically conservative, heteronormative theory that is no longer helpful and relevant for political struggles with regard to sexuality continues in contemporary feminist and queer literature.

For obvious reasons, *Three Essays* is a crucial text in the ongoing discussion on the status of Freudian thought and its relation to sexual politics. *Three Essays* does indeed contain a new theory of sexuality that undermines every pathologizing and moralistic approach to it. More particularly, *Three Essays* studies human sexuality from the perspective of the perversions; that is, from the perspective of what psychiatry had called sexual "aberrations." The study of the perversions allows us to determine the partial drives and the erogenous zones that form the building blocks of sexuality. These building blocks are present from the very beginning of our existence. Freud defines infantile sexuality as intrinsically polymorphous perverse. In the first edition of his text, he does not prioritize the different erogenous zones that constitute it, but rather speaks of a "need for variation" that characterizes human sexuality. This means that there is no essential primacy of genital sexuality that would be inscribed in the very nature of sexuality as such. Infantile sexuality is not in search of an object; it is only interested in pleasure. According to Freud, infantile sexuality is indeed essentially autoerotic. Not mediated by phantasy, it can be described in purely physiological terms. The relative importance of the different erogenous zones in adult life is thus the effect of (contingent) fixations of previous pleasurable bodily experiences. Freudian sexuality is not essentially phallocentric, let alone heteronormative.

One of the central aspects of Freud's *Three Essays* consists of a radically new perspective on the distinction between "pathology" and "normality." Pathology and normality can no longer be thought of as mutually exclusive. They are not essentially, but only gradually, different from one another. What is "pathological" is nothing less and nothing more than an exaggeration of what is normal, and what is normal is nothing but a diminished version of the pathological. There is no essential difference between the two. In this way, Freud criticizes the psychiatric idea that there exist "perverse identities" that can be described as such. Freud breaks away from the "psychiatric style of reasoning." This has far-reaching political consequences beyond the realm of psychiatry, notably with regard to the status of the perversions. Even in those instances where Freud does distinguish sexual pathology from sexual normality, he refuses to essentialize them. Every society distinguishes what is allowed from what is not. This idea should be linked to the spontaneous installation of reaction formations in every one of us. In contemporary Western societies, this distinction is to a large extent replaced by a distinction between what is "pathological" and what is not. But there are no foundations in sexuality itself that would justify this distinction once and for all. The latter has no *fundamentum in re*.

Freud is an anti-Aristotelian. That we call a certain type of behavior "pathology" largely depends on historical and social circumstances, not on the very essence of sexuality (Freud 1905d: 50). This idea also justifies the psychoanalytic critique of bourgeois sexual morality.

Is Freud, then, a queer theorist *avant la lettre*? Again, one should be cautious not to draw conclusions too fast. Even if the perspective we just developed largely dominates the first parts of the first edition of *Three Essays*, it is succeeded by a much more heteronormative approach in the third essay. In the later editions and in other texts focusing on the perversions, such as "A Child is Being Beaten" (Freud 1919b), Freud defends the position that the history of the development of the relations to the parents is decisive for the psychological identity and integration of the partial drives under the primacy of genitality. The partial drives are now situated on a developmental line that is grounded in the very nature of psychosexuality and that needs to be respected. This complex psychological process ideally leads to the institution of a male or female position that is in agreement with one's biological sex. These positions are, in other words, once again understood in heterosexual terms. What was previously called a "poetic fable" now threatens to become the obligatory outcome of psychological development (Haute 2002).

What this means for the perversions can be illustrated by the case of the theory of fetishism. In his late work, Freud links perversion – and more specifically fetishism – to the traumatic confrontation with sexual difference (the castration of the mother). The little child defends itself against this traumatic experience by denying it, which in turn leads to a splitting of the ego (Freud 1927, 1940). According to Freud, the creation of a fetish implies both the denial and the recognition of castration. This splitting is often manifest in the choice of a fetish that combines both aspects or in an attitude toward the fetish that is addressed both aggressively (recognition) and tenderly (denial). In short, the origin of a perversion – fetishism, for instance – is linked to an "abnormal" ("traumatic") moment; that is to say, it can be described in terms of an "abnormal" reaction to the threat of castration with which every child in its psychic development is confronted. The perversion is then once again an "aberration" from a normal development. The psychiatric style of reasoning takes over once again.

In more general terms, we can say that as a result of the introduction of the Oedipus complex, the perversions tend to be understood as developmental disorders (Lantéri-Laura 2012). This neutralizes the radical consequences of the first edition of *Three Essays*. The sexual perversions are now interpreted as aberrations and distortions; that is, as specific results of a "failed" history. In this way they are linked once again to specific identities. This return of the "psychiatric style of reasoning" implies a redefinition of sexuality. Sexuality is no longer understood in terms of nonfunctional bodily pleasures; these pleasures are now subordinated to a heterosexual norm that determines sexuality's value and significance. Sexuality once again will be defined in terms of knowledge of sexual difference (based on the earliest perceptions of the genital organs) and the sexual life of children and adults in terms of its psychic implications. This means that the various pleasures are made suspect again, as they become the markers of perverse – socially and morally problematic – inclinations. Behind the psychiatric style of reasoning one can detect the long Western tradition of a moral problematization of sexual pleasure and the gradual emergence of biopolitics in modernity, as clearly shown by Foucault in his *History of Sexuality*.

With regard to sexual politics, and notably the perversions, Freudian thinking is characterized by a tension between the two tendencies we have already mentioned – a more liberatory and a more conservative one. Many, if not most, post-Freudian scholars and practitioners joined up with the second tendency. The normalizing tendencies gained the upper hand in many post-Freudian writings and in psychoanalytic practice. They are still dominant in many psychoanalytic quarters today (Tort 2005: 423–434). Many post-Freudians consider the perversions once again psychic identities that can be differentiated from one another and from what is considered (heterosexual) "normality." In contradistinction to Freud, they also link perversion in general – and not just sadism and masochism – with aggressive and destructive tendencies. They cling to the idea that sexual perversion constitutes a specific diagnostic and psychological human "kind" (Hacking 2004) in which sexual life gets hijacked by destructive goals or hatred as the opposite of love (Carveth 2010: 300). All these authors underline the defensive meaning of the perversions (Stoller 1975; Chasseguet-Smirgel 1984a, 1984b). The American psychoanalyst Robert Stoller, who is a central voice in this debate, describes perversion as an eroticized form of hatred that is a response to a traumatic experience (Stoller 1975). The perverted act aims at hurting the other, not loving them (Ibid.: 97). According to Janine Chasseguet-Smirgel, perversion is characterized by a negation of the "paternal universe," of which the acceptation of sexual difference (castration) and the difference between the generations are the central features (Chasseguet-Smirgel 1984a). She further links perversion with a regression to the anal phase (Chasseguet-Smirgel 1978), whose importance is also recognized by other authors (Kernberg 1997). According to Chasseguet-Smirgel, this regression explains the perfidy and tendencies toward idealization and destructivity that are intrinsic parts of the pervert identity (Chasseguet-Smirgel 1984a: 185ff, 1984b; Whitebook 1991). In this regard, Otto Kernberg writes: "[f]rom a descriptive viewpoint, perversions can be classified along a continuum of severity, according to the degree to which aggression dominates a particular perversion" (Kernberg 2006: 22).[4]

It does not come as a surprise, then, that these authors, in contradiction to Freud, describe the perversions in negative terms, and that they consider sadism to be their ultimate paradigm (Whitebook 1991). Ever since the work of Augustine, the Western (religious) tradition linked the sexual perversions to evil. These perversions were considered evil because they did not respect a God-given order that forever links sexuality to procreation (Haute & Westerink 2017). Perversions go against nature and as such also go against the law of God. Freud – as well as the sexologists of his time – dismisses this tradition. In Freud's early texts, perversion is just a fixation to a specific form of pleasure; and since a hierarchy of pleasures would not make sense, he does not disqualify perverted pleasures. As discussed previously, in his later work, Freud replaces the teleological tradition with a psychiatric one. Perversions are now considered pathologies again, but they are not rejected as morally wrong. The post-Freudians, by contrast, tend to (re)combine the psychiatric approach with a (at least implicit) moral rejection. They consider perversion intrinsically destructive and for that reason link it to evil once again. Jacques Lacan and his followers identify a perverse structure.[5] This structure – distinguished from a psychotic and a neurotic structure – defines a specific subjective position characterized by a systematic undermining of society as such (Dean 2008). Indeed, according to Lacan, the perverse subject both acknowledges and denies the fundamental law that founds human society. Depending on context, Lacan associates this law with the law of the father, the law of sexual difference, or the law of castration. This law ("no") of the father (that separates us from the first Other, the Mother) inherently refers to the interdiction of incest or to the obligation of exogamy (and hence to the law of sexual difference) that founds the human order. Consequently, the perverse subject does not question this or that specific law. On the contrary, it actively subverts the order of legality as such.[6] Hence, we can understand the negative attitude of many Lacanian psychoanalysts toward the perversions.[7] Indeed, this negative attitude hardly comes as a surprise when we realize that the perversions are defined as a direct threat to the very existence of human society.[8] Insofar as the traditional (sexual) perversions continue to have a paradigmatic value within the so-called perverse structure, their negative qualification (and the rejection implied by it) and moral rejection also remain intact (or are reinstated).[9]

It is important to realize that Lacan (and, even more so, his string of followers) considers these structures to be in principle mutually exclusive. It is precisely for this reason that they resemble diagnostic identities. The Freudian patho-analytic perspective points toward an alternative that does not involve fixated "structures" and identities, but rather a network of associated psychic dynamics and issues. This is what Freud will call a complex. In hysteria, he finds the complex that allows us to gain a deeper insight into sexuality. This complex evolves around the excitable body, the autoerotic pleasures and perverse tendencies, and shame and disgust. This was articulated, as we know, in *Three Essays*. The study of obsessional neurosis confronts Freud with the Oedipus complex, which describes the interactions between the relation to authority, aggression, identification, conscience, and guilt formations. Narcissism, as well as the problems related to the ego in its relation to outside reality, is mainly linked to the study of the psychoses. And melancholia, finally, reveals a complex evolving around loss, love, identification, self-reproach, and death. The various psychopathologies show in a magnified and exaggerated way psychic dynamics that, according to Freud, can be considered generally human. That means that these complexes are not mutually exclusive but partly overlapping; they help us understand human psychic life and existence. From a patho-analytic perspective, the various complexes are present in all of us and have a "universal" status, but they play a truly determining role in *only one* specific pathology. A patho-analytic perspective thus, at least potentially, offers an alternative to a theory of mutually exclusive structures and identities.

There are occasions where Freud goes even further and links these psychopathologies to different cultural phenomena. In *Totem and Taboo*, for instance, he writes:

> [t]he neuroses exhibit on the one hand striking and far-reaching points of agreement with those great social institutions, art, religion and philosophy. But on the other hand they seem like distortions of them. It might be maintained that a case of hysteria is a caricature of a work of art, that an obsessional neurosis is a caricature of a religion and that a paranoiac delusion is a caricature of a philosophical system.
>
> *(Freud 1912–13: 73)*

Not only do the psychopathologies inform us about the fundamentals of human existence, but they also have a privileged relation to crucial cultural formations: art, religion, and philosophy – that is, those cultural phenomena that cannot be explained in functional terms, i.e., as being in service of self-preservation or preservation of the species. This does not mean that these cultural phenomena are pathologies; it means that these phenomena can be studied from the perspective of the psychopathologies, as they show – in a magnified way – analogous "complexes." This does not mean that, for Freud, culture could ever replace "pathology." There are no firm solutions to the typical human problems we discover through studying the pathologies at hand. Every answer is provisional and incomplete: in cultural formations, the conflicts and tensions characterizing psychic life are continued. It follows that the human being is a "being-of-the-in-between": humans realize their existence in a constant and irresolvable tension between pathology and culture (Haute & Geyskens 2012).

Freud did not consistently and fully develop this patho-analytic line of reasoning. His fascination for the Oedipus complex as the "nucleus of all neuroses" (Freud 1912–13: 157) and the subsequent role he gave it in his metapsychology made this impossible. Instead of radically pursuing a patho-analytic approach to psychic life and culture, Freud pushed toward the primacy of one complex that, linked with a developmental approach to psychic life and culture, progressively moved toward a theory that "ideally" described the so-called normal "dissolution of the Oedipus complex" (Freud 1924b). In this way, psychoanalysis could become a "normalization" machine that defined the "normal" outcome of sexual development in a heterosexual organization of sexual life while pressing the "abnormal" perverse activities into the margins of existence. The idea of normalization and its accompanying "repression," however, runs counter to some of Freud's basic and most productive intuitions.

This short overview of post-Freudian thinking on the perversions, structures, and identities and their roots in elements of Freudian thought as well as the possibility of a Freudian critique shows Freud's thought to be potentially liberating and critical toward mechanisms of exclusion; at the same time, it has to be said that his critics were not mistaken in rejecting psychoanalysis's moralizing and heteronormative approach to (perverted) sexuality. What our rereading of Freud's *Three*

Essays shows is exactly this: psychoanalysis – in Freud's hands and even more so in the hands of a considerable number of his followers – developed from a potentially liberating theory into a strong support base for the heterosexual matrix. This became clear in our reading of *Three Essays*: from a radical critique of the psychiatric "poetic fable" about human sexuality, it gradually became a subtle defense of it in the later versions, especially from the third edition onward. But this also means that psychoanalysis cannot be reduced to an exponent of a history of the disciplinary domestication of pleasurable sexual activities that we find throughout the Western tradition (Foucault 1978). Psychoanalysis cannot be reduced to its oedipalized version. Instead, we have shown that Freud's early texts have a potential for subverting this oedipal version from within. After all, in the 1905 *Three Essays*, primacy is not accorded to the object, but to the excitable body, as a source of pleasure. This fact cannot but remind us of "the body of pleasures" invoked by Foucault at the end of the first volume of his *History of Sexuality* as a critical reference point against all forms of sexual (oedipal) normalization (Foucault 1978: 159). We know that Freud explored these pleasures from the perspective of the perversions. In so doing, he inevitably took his starting point in the psychiatric tradition that Foucault is criticizing. But Freud only did so to undermine and problematize the very idea of "perversions" as specific psychological identities (Davidson 2001).

In this context, Freud is on Foucault's side. Moreover, Freud's "patho-analytic approach" is also undoubtedly relevant for contemporary discussions, not on account of a simple application of the models and "complexes" identified by him but by virtue of a consequent patho-analytic deconstruction of identities and identity markers. In *Three Essays*, Freud takes homosexuality as a starting point to defend the contingent character of the sexual object and sexual activities. This did not prevent Freud, however, from thinking about sexuality in binary terms. This is quite obvious in his later work, in which the Oedipus complex is meant to establish a male and female position that, at least in principle, can be strictly held apart. His concept of bisexuality in the earlier writings is likewise conceived from the perspective of two poles – "male" and "female" – that remain strictly distinct, even if they are combined "positions" in every human being. One could now pursue a patho-analytic approach that starts from transgenderism, for instance, to further deconstruct fundamental Freudian presuppositions with regard to sexuality that have become highly problematic for us (Gherovici 2017). Transgenderism was not much of an issue for Freud and his contemporaries (Davidson 2001), but nothing prevents us from further following Freud's fundamental intuition that the different sexual "identities" and orientations potentially inform us about fundamental characteristics and problematics of human sexuality as such. In this respect, it would be possible – and desirable – to write a fourth (contemporary) essay on the theory of sexuality, taking into account more recent problematics and "complexes," thus extending Freudian psychoanalysis beyond its historical limitations. It would be presumptuous to consider Freud a queer theorist *avant la lettre*, of course, but our reading and analysis of *Three Essays* show that he is certainly also not the heteronormative ideologist he is sometimes made out to be. On the contrary, for a contemporary psychoanalytic approach to a philosophical anthropology centered around the body as a source of pleasure, Freudian psychoanalysis remains an inevitable point of reference not to be overlooked.

Notes

1 Compare also the preparatory remarks to the Dora case where Freud draws an analogy between psychoanalytic analyses and reconstructions and the work of archaeologists (Freud 1905d: 12).
2 However, such narrative in principle seems at odds with a psychoanalytic theory and practice that fundamentally question unity, coherence, and consistency in both the speaker and his or her narrative.
3 "The author is therefore the ideological figure by which one marks the manner in which we fear the proliferation of meaning" (Foucault 1984: 119).
4 In this context, one could also think of Melanie Klein, for whom perversion is a schizoid identity problem that is further linked to the vicissitudes of the death drive (Roudinesco 2014; Hinshelwood 1994).
5 For a more detailed account of the Lacanian approach in relation to the positions on the perversions we just mentioned, see Haute 2016.
6 In this respect, Stephanie Swales writes: "[t]he perverse subject is he who has undergone alienation but disavowed castration, suffering from excessive *jouissance* and a core belief that the law and social norms are fraudulent at worse and weak at best" (Swales 2012: xii).
7 For illustrations, see Haute 2016.
8 What should also be considered in this context is the influence of French psychiatrist Ernest Dupré on Lacan's theory of the perversions. Dupré was a contemporary of Lacan's "master in psychiatry," Clérambault. Dupré determined French psychiatric thinking on the perversions from the early 1920s until at least 1960. He reintroduced a highly moralizing and dismissive attitude toward the perversions into French psychiatric thinking. For Dupré's influence on Lacan and references, see Haute 2016.
9 We should indeed remember that classical sexology tried to get rid of these negative qualifications by claiming that the perversions were mental illnesses and escaped our free will. The corresponding attitude has been that perverted subjects deserve our help and attention, not rejection.

BIBLIOGRAPHY

Abraham, K. (1908). Die psychosexuellen Differenzen der Hysterie und der Dementia Praecox, in *Psychoanalytische Studien, Band II*, Gießen: Psychosozial-Verlag, 132–145.

Adler, A. (1908). Der Aggressionstrieb im Leben und in der Neurose, in *Fortschritte der Medizin* 26, 577–584.

Beer, M.D. (1995). Psychosis: From Mental Disorder to Disease Concept, in *History of Psychiatry* 6(2), 177–200.

Bernet, R. (2013). *Force-pulsion-désir. Une autre philosophie de la psychanalyse*, Paris: Vrin.

Binet, A. (1887). Le fétichisme dans l'amour, in *Revue Philosophique* 24, 142–167.

Binswanger, L. (1920). Psychoanalyse und klinische Psychiatrie, in *Ausgewählte Vorträge und Aufsätze, Band II. Zur Problematik der psychiatrischen Forschung und zum Problem der Psychiatrie*, Bern: Francke Verlag, 1955.

Binswanger, O. (1904). *Die Hysterie*, Vienna: Alfred Hölder.

Blass, R. (1992). Did Dora have an Oedipus Complex? A Re-examination of the Theoretical Context of Freud's 'Fragment of an Analysis', in *Psychoanalytic Study of the Child* 47, 159–187.

Blass, R. (2017). Understanding Freud's Conflicted View of the Object-relatedness of Sexuality and its Implications for Contemporary Psychoanalysis: A Re-examination of *Three Essays on the Theory of Sexuality*, in Ph. Van Haute & H. Westerink (Eds.), *Deconstructing Normativity? Freud's 1905 Three Essays*, New York/London: Routledge, 6–27.

Bleuler, E. (1916). *Lehrbuch der Psychiatrie*, Berlin: Springer.

Bloch, I. (1902). *Beiträge zur Aetiologie der Psychopathia sexualis*, Dresden: Dohrn.

Borch-Jacobsen, M. (1982). *Le sujet freudien*, Paris: Flammarion.

Bowlby, J. (1969). *Attachment and Loss*, New York: Basic Books.

Butler, J. (1999). Revisiting Bodies and Pleasures, in *Theory, Culture & Society* 16(2), 11–20.

Carveth, D. (2010). How Today May We Distinguish Healthy Sexuality from "Perversion"? in *Canadian Journal of Psychoanalysis/Revue canadienne de psychanalyse* 18(2), 296–305.

Chasseguet-Smirgel, J. (1978). Reflexions on the Connexions between Perversion and Sadism, in *International Journal of Psychoanalysis* 59(1), 27–37.

Chasseguet-Smirgel, J. (1984a). *Ethique et esthétique de la perversion*, Seyssel: Champ Vallon.

Chasseguet-Smirgel, J. (1984b). *The Ego Ideal. A Psychoanalytic Essay on the Maladie of the Ideal*, London/New York: Norton.

Darwin, Ch. (1981). *The Descent of Man, and Selection in Relation to Sex*, with an introduction by J.T. Bonner & R.M. May, Princeton: Princeton University Press.

Davidson, A.I. (1984). Assault on Freud, in *London Review of Books* 6(12), 9–11.

Davidson, A.I. (2001). *The Emergence of Sexuality: Historical Epistemology and the Formation of Concepts*, Cambridge, MA: Harvard University Press.

De Block, A. (2004). *De vogel van Leonardo. Freuds opvattingen over de relatie tussen seksualiteit, cultuur en psychische gezondheid*, Leuven: Acco.

De Vleminck, J. (2013). *De schaduw van Kaïn. Freuds klinische antropologie van de agressiviteit*, Leuven: Universitaire Pers.

De Vleminck, J. (2017). Freud reads Krafft-Ebing: The Case of Sadism and Masochism, in Ph. Van Haute & H. Westerink (Eds.), *Deconstructing Normativity? Freud's 1905 Three Essays*, New York/London: Routledge, 64–86.

Dean, T. (2001). Homosexuality and the Problem of Otherness, in T. Dean & Chr. Lane (Eds.), *Homosexuality & Psychoanalysis*, Chicago: Chicago University Press, 120–143.

Dean, T. (2008). The Frozen Countenance of Perversion, in *Parallax* 14(2), 93–114.

Deleuze, G. & Guattari, F. (1972). *Anti-Oedipus. Capitalism and Schizophrenia*, New York: Viking Press, 1977.

Ellis, H. (1900). *Studies in the Psychology of Sex*, Vol. 1, Philadelphia/London: Davis Publishers, 1918.

Falzeder, E. (2007). The Story of an Ambivalent Relationship: Sigmund Freud and Eugen Bleuler, in *Journal of Analytical Psychology* 52(3), 343–368.

Finzi, D. & Westerink, H. (Eds.) (2018). *Dora – Hysteria – Gender. Reconsidering Freud's Case Study. A Sigmund Freud Museum's Symposium*, Leuven: Leuven University Press.

Fletcher, J. (2013). *Freud and the Scene of Trauma*, New York: Fordham University Press.

Foucault, M. (1978). *The History of Sexuality, Vol. 1: An Introduction*, New York: Pantheon Books.

Foucault, M. (1984). What is an Author? in P. Rabinow (Ed.), *Foucault Reader*, New York: Pantheon Books.

Foucault, M. (1985). *The History of Sexuality, Vol. 2: The Use of Pleasure*, New York: Pantheon Books.

Foucault, M. (2018). *Histoire de la sexualité 4: Les aveux de la chair*, Paris: Éditions Gallimard.

Freud, S. (1890). Psychical (or Mental) Treatment, in J. Strachey (Ed.), *Standard Edition (SE)* 7, London: Hogarth.

Freud, S. (1893). On the Psychical Mechanism of Hysterical Phenomena: Preliminary Communication, *SE 2*.

Freud, S. (1894). The Neuro-Psychoses of Defence, *SE 3*.

Freud, S. (1895). On the Grounds for Detaching a Particular Syndrome from Neurasthenia under the Description "Anxiety Neurosis", *SE 3*.

Freud, S. (1896a). Extracts from the Fliess Papers (Draft K), *SE 1*.

Freud, S. (1896b). The Aetiology of Hysteria, *SE 1*.

Freud, S. (1898). Sexuality in the Aetiology of the Neuroses, *SE 3*.

Freud, S. (1900). *The Interpretation of Dreams, SE 4–5*.

Freud, S. (1905a). *Three Essays on the Theory of Sexuality. The 1905 Edition*, Ph. Van Haute, U. Kistner & H. Westerink (Eds.), New York/London: Verso, 2016.

Freud, S. (1905b). *Jokes and their Relation to the Unconscious, SE 8*.

Freud, S. (1905c). *Three Essays on the Theory of Sexuality, SE 7*.

Freud, S. (1905d). Fragment of an Analysis of a Case of Hysteria, *SE 7*.

Freud, S. (1906). My Views on the Part Played by Sexuality in the Aetiology of the Neuroses, *SE 7*.

Freud, S. (1907). Obsessive Acts and Religious Practices, *SE 9*.

Freud, S. (1908a). On the Sexual Theories of Children, *SE 9*.

Freud, S. (1908b). "Civilized" Sexual Ethics and Modern Nervous Illness, *SE 9*.

Freud, S. (1908c). Creative Writers and Day-Dreaming, *SE 9*.

Freud, S. (1909a). Analysis of a Phobia in a Five-Year-Old Boy, *SE 10*.

Freud, S. (1909b). Family Romances, *SE 9*.

Freud, S. (1909c). Notes upon a Case of Obsessional Neurosis, *SE 10*.

Freud, S. (1910a). *Five Lectures on Psycho-Analysis, SE 11*.

Freud, S. (1910b). *Leonardo da Vinci and a Memory of his Childhood, SE 11*.

Freud, S. (1911). Psychoanalytic Remarks on an Autobiographically Described Case of Paranoia (Dementia paranoids), *SE 12*.

Freud, S. (1912). The Dynamics of Transference, *SE 12*.

Freud, S. (1912–1913). *Totem and Taboo, SE 13*.

Freud, S. (1913). The Disposition to Obsessional Neurosis, *SE 12*.

Freud, S. (1914a). On Narcissism: An Introduction, *SE 14*.

Freud, S. (1914b). On the History of the Psycho-Analytic Movement, *SE 14*.

Freud, S. (1914c). Remembering, Repeating and Working-Through, *SE 12*.

Freud, S. (1915). Instincts and their Vicissitudes, *SE 14*.

Freud, S. (1916). On Transience, *SE 14*.

Freud, S. (1917). Mourning and Melancholia, *SE 14*.

Freud, S. (1918). From the History of an Infantile Neurosis, *SE 17*.

Freud, S. (1919a). Introduction to *Psychoanalysis and the War Neuroses, SE 17*.

Freud, S. (1919b). A Child is Being Beaten, *SE 17*.

Freud, S. (1920). *Beyond the Pleasure Principle, SE 18*.

Freud, S. (1921). *Group Psychology and the Analysis of the Ego, SE 18*.

Freud, S. (1923a). The Infantile Genital Organization of the Libido, *SE 19*.

Freud, S. (1923b). *The Ego and the Id, SE 19*.

Freud, S. (1924a). The Economic Problem of Masochism, *SE 19*.

Freud, S. (1924b). The Dissolution of the Oedipus Complex, *SE 19*.

Freud, S. (1925). An Autobiographical Study, *SE 20*.

Freud, S. (1927). Fetishism, *SE 21*.

Freud, S. (1930). *Civilization and its Discontents, SE 21*.

Freud, S. (1940). The Splitting of the Ego and in the Process of Defence, *SE 23*.

Freud, S. (1950). Project for a Scientific Psychology, *SE 1*.

Freud, S. (1985). *The Complete Letters of Sigmund Freud to Wilhelm Fliess 1887–1904*, Cambridge/London: Harvard University Press.

Freud, S. (2005). *Drei Abhandlungen zur Sexualtheorie*, with an introduction by R. Reiche, Frankfurt: Fischer.

Freud, S. (2015). *Drei Abhandlungen zur Sexualtheorie (1905)*, Ph. Van Haute, Chr. Huber & H. Westerink (Eds.), Sigmund Freuds Werke – Wiener Interdisziplinäre Kommentare, Band 2, Vienna: Vienna University Press.

Freud, S. (2017). *Drie verhandelingen over de theorie van de seksualiteit (1905)*, Ph. Van Haute & H. Westerink (Eds.), Nijmegen: Vantilt.

Fuchs, A. (1902). Therapeutische Bestrebungen auf dem Gebiete sexueller Perversionen, in *Jahrbuch für sexuelle Zwischenstufen* 4, 177–186.

Gay, P. (1988). *Freud. A Life for our Times*, New York: Norton.

Geyskens, T. (2005). *Our Original Scenes: Freud's theory of Sexuality*, Leuven: Leuven University Press.

Gherovici, P. (2017). *Transgender Psychoanalysis*, New York: Routledge.

Hacking, I. (2004). Making up People, in *Historical Ontology*, Cambridge, MA: Harvard University Press, 99–114.

Haute, Ph. Van (2002). The Introduction of the Oedipus Complex and the Re-invention of Instinct. Freud's 'Three Essays on the Theory of Sexuality', in *Radical Philosophy* 115, 7–15.

Haute, Ph. Van (2005). Psychoanalysis and/as Philosophy: The Anthropological Significance of Pathology in Freud's Three Essays on the Theory of Sexuality and in the Psychoanalytic Tradition, in *Natureza Humana* 7(2), 359–374.

Haute, Ph. Van (2013). Het project van een pathoanalyse van het bestaan in Freuds *Drie verhandelingen over de theorie van de seksualiteit*, in Ph. Van Haute & J. De Vleminck (Eds.), *Freud als filosoof: Over seksualiteit, psychopathologie en cultuur*, Kalmthout: Pelckmans, 33–49.

Haute, Ph. Van (2016). Lacan Meets Freud? Patho-Analytic Reflections on the Status of the Perversions in Lacanian Metapsychology, in *Studies in Gender and Sexuality* 17(4), 274–284.

Haute, Ph. Van (2018). Trauma and Disgust. Dora between Freud and Laplanche, in D. Finzi & H. Westerink (Eds.), *Dora – Hysteria – Gender. Reconsidering Freud's Case Study. A Sigmund Freud Museum's Symposium*, Leuven: Leuven University Press, 59–72.

Haute, Ph. Van & Geyskens, T. (2004). *Confusion of Tongues: The Primacy of Sexuality in Freud, Ferenczi and Laplanche*, New York: Other Press.

Haute, Ph. Van & Geyskens, T. (2012). *A Non-Oedipal Psychoanalysis? A Clinical Anthropology of Hysteria in the Work of Freud and Lacan*, Leuven: Leuven University Press.

Haute, Ph. Van & Geyskens, T. (2016). Wut, Wollust und Wankelmut. Eine freudianische Symptomatologie der Zwangsneurose, in *Zeitschrift: texte – psychoanalyse. ästhetik. kulturkritik* 36(4), 11–26.

Haute, Ph. Van, Kistner, U. & Westerink, H. (2017). Freud vertalen, Freud verraden? Over de vertaling van 'Trieb' in de *Drie verhandelingen over de theorie van de seksualiteit*, in *Tijdschrift voor psychoanalyse* 23(3), 186–197.

Haute, Ph. Van & Westerink, H. (2016a). Sexuality and Its Object in Freud's 1905 Edition of 'Three Essays on the Theory of Sexuality', in *International Journal of Psychoanalysis* 97(3), 563–589.

Haute, Ph. Van & Westerink, H. (2016b). Hysterie, Sexualität und die Dekonstruktion der Normativität. Eine Relektüre der ersten Ausgabe von Freud "Drei Abhandlungen zur Sexualtheorie", in *Psyche-Zeitschrift für Psychoanalyse und ihre Anwendungen* 70(3), 212–250.

Haute, Ph. Van & Westerink, H. (Eds.) (2017). *Deconstructing Normativity? Freud's 1905 Three Essays*, New York/London: Routledge.

Haute, Ph. Van & Westerink, H. (2020). 'Family Romances' and the Oedipalization of Freudian Psychoanalysis, in *Psychoanalysis and History* 22(2), 175–187.

Hinshelwood, R.D. (1994). *Clinical Klein*, London: Free Association Books.

Hirschfeld, M. (1899). Die objective Diagnose der Homosexualität, in *Jahrbuch für sexuelle Zwischenstufen* 1.

Jaspers, K. (1913). *Allgemeine Psychopathologie*, Berlin: Springer.

Jung, C.G. (1907). *Uber die Psychologie der Dementia Praecox. Ein Versuch*, Halle: Verlagsbuchhandlung Carl Marhold.

Jung, C.G. (1912a). *Psychology of the Unconscious*, Mineola, NY: Dover Publications, 2002.

Jung, C.G. (1912b). Versuch einer Darstellung der psychoanaltischen Theorie, in *Gesammelte Werke* 4, Solothurn: Walter Verlag, 107–255.

Kernberg, O. (2006). Perversion, Perversity and Normality: Diagnostic and Therapeutic Considerations' (1997), in D. Nobus & L. Downing (Eds.), *Perversion. Psychoanalytic perspectives /Perspectives on Psychoanalysis*, London: Karnac Books, 19–38.

Kloocke, R., Schmiedebach, H.-P. & Priebe, S. (2005). Psychological Injury in the two World Wars: Changing Concepts and Terms in German Psychiatry, in *History of Psychiatry* 16(1), 43–60.

Kraepelin, E. (1915). *Psychiatrie. Ein Lehrbuch für Studierende und Ärzte, Band 4 (Teil 3)*, Leipzig: Barth.

Krafft-Ebing, R. von (1886). *Psychopathia Sexualis, with Especial Reference to the Antipathic Sexual Instinct: A Medico-Forensic Study*, F.E. Klaf (Ed.), New York: Arcade Publishing, 1965.

Krafft-Ebing, R. von (1901). Neue Studien auf dem Gebiete der Homosexualität, in *Jahrbuch für sexuelle Zwischenstufen* 3, 1–36.

Kris, E. (1952). Einleitung zur Erstausgabe, in *Sigmund Freud. Briefe an Wilhelm Fließ*, Frankfurt: Fischer, 1986.

Lacan, J. (1966). *Écrits*, Paris: Seuil.

Lantéri-Laura, G. (2012). *Lecture des Perversions: Histoire de Leur Appropriation Médical*, Paris: Economica/Anthropos.

Laplanche, J. (1976). *Life and Death in Psychoanalysis*, with an introduction by J. Mehlman, Baltimore/London: The John Hopkins University Press.

Laplanche, J. (1987). *Nouveaux fondements pour la psychanalyse*, Paris: Presses Universitaires de France.

Laplanche, J. (1992). The Freud Museum Seminar (3 May 1990), in J. Fletcher & M. Stanton (Eds.), *Seduction, Translation, Drives*, London: Psychoanalytic Forum/Institute of Contemporary Arts.

Laplanche, J. (2006). *L'après-coup (Problématiques VI)*, Paris: Presses Universitaires de France.

Laplanche, J. (2007). *Sexual. La sexualité élargie au sens freudien*, Paris: Presses Universitaires de France.

Lear, J. (2005). *Freud*, New York/London: Routledge.

Lerner, P. (2003). *Hysterical Men, War, Psychiatry, and the Politics of Trauma in Germany, 1890–1930*, Ithaca: Cornell University Press.

Marcuse, H. (1955). *Eros and Civilisation. A Philosophical Inquiry into Freud*, Boston: Beacon Press.

Marder, E. (2015). L'Homme aux loups. L'animal sexuel et la scène primitive, in G. Ribault (Ed.), *Freud au cas par cas. Lectures philosophiques des cas freudiens*, Leuven: Leuven University Press, 127–148.

Marinelli, L. & Mayer, A. (2003). *Dreaming by the Book. A History of Freud's "Interpretation of Dreams" and the Psychoanalytic Movement*, New York: Other Press.

Martins, V. (2019). *L'Oedipe selon Foucault. Foucault lecteur et non-lecteur de Freud à travers le 'complexe d'Oedipe'*, non-published PhD-thesis (dir. L. Laufer and A. Vanier): Université Paris Diderot.

Masson, J. (1984). *Assault on Truth. Freud's Suppression of the Seduction Theory*, New York: Farrar, Straus and Giroux.

May-Tolzmann, U. (1998). 'Obsessional Neurosis': A Nosographic Innovation by Freud, in *History of Psychiatry* 9(3), 335–353.

May-Tolzmann, U. (2015a). *Freud bei der Arbeit. Zur Entstehungsgeschichte der psychoanalytischen Theorie und Praxis, mit der Auswertung von Freuds Patientenkalender*, Gießen: Psychosozial-Verlag.

May-Tolzmann, U. (2015b). The Third Step in Drive Theory: On the Genesis of Beyond the Pleasure Principle, in *Psychoanalysis and History* 17(2), 205–272.

Mazaleigue, J. (2014). *Les déséquilibres de l'amour: la genèse du concept de perversion sexuelle, de la revolution française à Freud*, Paris: Ithaque.

Meyer, A. (2016). *Sigmund Freud. Zur Einführung*, Hamburg: Junius.

Micale, M. (1993). On the 'Disappearance' of Hysteria. A Study in the Clinical Deconstruction of a Diagnosis, in *Isis* 84(3), 496–526.

Moll, A. (1898). *Untersuchungen über die Libido sexualis, Bd*, Vol. 1, Berlin: Fischer.

Moyaert, P. (1994). *Ethiek en sublimatie*, Nijmegen: Socialistische Uitgeverij Nijmegen.

Moyaert, P. (2012). Seksualiteit is niet te integreren: Hoe Freud over de "conditio humana" nadenkt, in *Filosofie* 22(4), 2–14.

Moyaert, P. (2014). *Opboksen tegen het inerte. De doodsdrift bij Freud*, Nijmegen: Van Tilt.

Müller-Funk, W. (2016). Das Unbehagen in der Kultur: Close Reading und Rezeptionsgeschichte, in W. Müller-Funk (Ed.), *S. Freud, Das Unbehagen in der Kultur*, Vienna: Vienna University Press, 7–45.

Nunberg, H. & Federn, E. (Eds.) (1962). *Minutes of the Vienna Psychoanalytic Society*, Vol. 3, New York: International Universities Press.

Oosterhuis, H. (2000). *Stepchildren of Nature: Krafft-Ebing, Psychiatry, and the Making of Sexual Identity*, Chicago: University of Chicago Press.

Oosterhuis, H. (2012). Sexual Modernity in the Works of Richard von Krafft-Ebing and Albert Moll, in *Medical History* 56(2), 133–155.

Phillips, A. (2014). *Becoming Freud. The Making of a Psychoanalyst*, New Haven/London: Yale University Press.

Quindeau, I. (2014). *Sexualität*, Gießen: Psychsozial-Verlag.

Quinodoz, J.-M. (2005). *Reading Freud. A Chronological Exploration of Freud's Writings*, New York: Routledge.

Rank, O. & Sachs, H. (1912). Entwicklung und Ansprüche der Psychoanalyse, in *Imago* 1, 1–16.

Roudinesco, E. (2014). *Sigmund Freud en son temps et dans le nôtre*, Paris: Seuil.

Sauerteig, L. (2012). Loss of Innocence: Albert Moll, Sigmund Freud and the Invention of Childhood Sexuality around 1900, in *Medical History* 56(2), 156–183.

Schotte, J. (1990). *Szondi avec Freud. Sur la voie d'une psychiatrie pulsionelle*, Bruxelles: Editions universitaires De Boeck.

Schröter, M. (Ed.) (2012). *Sigmund Freud – Eugen Bleuler: Ich bin zuversichtlich, wir erobern bald die Psychiatrie. Briefwechsel 1904–1937*, Basel: Schwabe.

Scull, A. (2009). Hysteria, in *The Disturbing History*, Oxford/New York: Oxford University Press.

Shorter, E. (1992). *From Paralysis to Fatigue: A History of Psychosomatic Illness in the Modern Era*, New York: Free Press.

Sigusch, V. (2012). The Sexologist Albert Moll – between Sigmund Freud and Magnus Hirschfeld, in *Medical History* 56(2), 184–200.

Spielrein, S. (1912). Die Destruktion als Ursache des Werdens, in *Sämtliche Schriften*, Freiburg: Verlag Traute Hensch, 98–143.

Stoller, R. (1975). *Perversion: The Erotic form of Hatred*, London: Karnac Books.

Sulloway, F. (1979). *Freud: Biologist of the Mind*, New York: Basic Books.

Swales, S. (2012). *Perversion: A Lacanian Psychoanalytic Approach to the Subject*, New York: Routledge.

Tort, M. (2005). *Fin du dogme paternel*, Paris: Aubier.

Vandermeersch, P. (1991). *Unresolved Questions in the Freud-Jung Debate on Psychosis, Sexual Identity and Religion*, Leuven: Leuven University Press.

Vandermeersch, P. (2017). The Mystery of the Erased Sentence in Freud's *Three Essays on the Theory of Sexuality*, in Ph. Van Haute & H. Westerink (Eds.), *Deconstructing Normativity? Freud's 1905 Three Essays*, New York/London: Routledge, 55–63.

Weber, M. (2015). Das Hysterie-Konzept der deutschen Psychiatrie um 1900 im Lehrbuch von Emil Kraepelin, in *Psychotherapie* 20(1), 50–64.

Westerink, H. (2009). *A Dark Trace: Sigmund Freud on the Sense of Guilt*, Leuven: Leuven University Press.

Westerink, H. (2014). Projection, Substitution and Exaltation: Freud's Case Study of Little Hans and the Creation of God in *Totem and Taboo*, in *Psychoanalysis and History* 16(1), 55–68.

Westerink, H. (2016). Der problematische Ort der Wut im Denken Freuds über Aggression, in *Zeitschrift: texte – psychoanalyse. ästhetik. kulturkritik* 36(4), 27–46.

Westerink, H. (2017). Eine Pathoanalyse der Religion. Bemerkungen zu einem unvollendeten Projekt Freuds, in *Wege zum Menschen* 69(4), 301–311.

Westerink, H. (2018). Sucking, Kissing and Disgust – Dora and Theory of Infantile Sexuality, in D. Finzi & H. Westerink (Eds.), *Dora – Hysteria – Gender. Reconsidering Freud's Case Study. A Sigmund Freud Museum's Symposium*, Leuven: Leuven University Press, 73–88.

Westerink, H. (2019). *De lichamen en hun lusten. In het spoor van Foucaults* Geschiedenis van de seksualiteit, Nijmegen: Vantilt.

Whitebook, J. (1991). Perversion: Destruction and Reparation. On the Contributions of Janine Chasseguet-Smirgel and Joyce McDougall, in *American Imago* 48(3), 329–350.

Woods, A. (2011). *The Sublime Object of Psychiatry: Schizophrenia in Clinical and Cultural Theory*, Oxford: Oxford University Press.

INDEX

For Product Safety Concerns and Information please contact our EU representative GPSR@taylorandfrancis.com
Taylor & Francis Verlag GmbH, Kaufingerstraße 24, 80331 München, Germany

www.ingramcontent.com/pod-product-compliance
Ingram Content Group UK Ltd.
Pitfield, Milton Keynes, MK11 3LW, UK
UKHW020207200926
475702UK00004B/658
9780367645304